Hacking Chemo

From the Marianne Williamson quote, long one of my favourites…

Our Deepest Fear

By Marianne Williamson

Our deepest fear is not that we are inadequate.
Our deepest fear is that we are powerful beyond measure.
It is our light, not our darkness
That most frightens us.
We ask ourselves
Who am I to be brilliant, gorgeous, talented, fabulous?
Actually, who are you not to be?
You are a child of God.
Your playing small
Does not serve the world.
There is nothing enlightened about shrinking
So that other people won't feel insecure around you.
We are all meant to shine,
As children do.
We were born to make manifest
The glory of God that is within us.
It's not just in some of us;
It's in everyone.
And as we let our own light shine,
We unconsciously give other people permission to do the same.
As we are liberated from our own fear,
Our presence automatically liberates others.

Used with permission. From: *A Return to Love*, Marianne Williamson, 1996.

Dedication

To all the powerful women and men who have been or will be blindsided by a cancer diagnosis. Take back your power!

And to Mike – my ROCK.

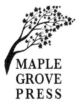

**MAPLE
GROVE
PRESS**

Maple Grove Press
PO Box 200015, Westside RO
Owen Sound ON
N4K 0E7

ISBN: 978-1-7771488-0-5 (print)
ISBN: 978-1-7771488-1-2(ebook)

Ordering Information:
Special discounts are available on quantity purchases by corporations, associations, and
others. For details, contact the author at martha@marthatettenborn.com

Table of Contents

Part 3: Practical Implementation

Part 4: Life Goes On...

Part 5: Easy Keto Recipes - Basics and Good Substitutes

Appendix 1: The Quick and Dirty Guide

Appendix 2: The Evidence /Research

Hacking Chemo

USING KETOGENIC DIET, THERAPEUTIC FASTING AND
A KICKASS ATTITUDE TO POWER THROUGH CANCER

MARTHA TETTENBORN RD

Disclaimer

Unlike many who write or preach dietary protocols, I *am* a health professional, with Registered Dietitian credentials behind my name. However, this book describes my *personal* journey using nutrition and lifestyle interventions to travel through the cancer treatment experience. As you, the reader, and I do not have a professional-to-patient relationship, this cannot be construed as a personalized nutritional prescription. If you or a loved one are facing cancer treatments and wish to use the interventions described in this book, you should discuss your plans with your medical team. There are some reasons that using a ketogenic diet or fasting as I have described may not be medically advised, and you need to listen to your medical team and ask for the reasons that you are being advised against this. See the chapter "When Keto and Fasting Are NOT Right for You." You may or may not get support from your medical team for your approach and, at that point, you need to take responsibility for your own health-impacting decisions. In the end, it's your journey…

Introduction

Cancer is a game-changer. No question.

When I found out I had cancer, I went looking for information. Not just research but experiences. I wanted to read and hear from other women who had been diagnosed with and treated for ovarian cancer. I wanted to find the ones diagnosed with stage 1C2 (self-contained, no abdominal tumour spread but ruptured in place). I wanted to find the ones who had a cyst. I wanted to hear from women my age. I wanted the nitty-gritty details of surgery, chemotherapy, radiation, side effects, strategies, interventions. I was hungry for others' stories. I was looking for hope, strategy, detail.

I wasn't yet ready to tell the world that I was now a "person with cancer," as I had to get my own head around it first. So I went to the internet, of course. But the internet tends to be a younger person's domain. I spent hours on YouTube watching videos entitled *My Ovarian Cancer Story*, or similar, but most of them were made by young women, in their twenties or thirties. They were informative but really didn't relate to *my* situation. Of course, this makes sense—young people who grew up comfortable with this technology were using it to put their stories online. But although ovarian cancer does affect women of all ages, the majority are over 50 years old and they simply weren't represented in the online world.

Boy oh boy, what I'd give to find someone in their fifties who could tell me their story…

At the same time, I was doing hours of online research into cancer itself: Watching lectures and educational videos from various institutions and conferences, reading articles on PubMed, and visiting the blogs and websites of a variety of prominent scientists and influencers in the field of cancer research and cancer treatment. And as I read, I became increasingly aware of the newly rediscovered field of cancer metabolism. Although the original research pointing to cancer as a disease of damaged metabolism had been carried out in the 1930s and won a Nobel Prize at the time, it had been spearheaded by a controversial German scientist who had the protection of the Nazi Party – despite being half Jewish. However, most things German were considered with low regard after the World Wars and Otto Warburg's research was forgotten. Add to that the cultural reality of Watson and Crick's discovery of DNA just a few years later—and the revelation that cancer had damaged genes as a hallmark feature—and off went the entire cancer establishment down the path of genetics, leaving metabolism to the dusty stacks of medical libraries.

Scientists have always known the metabolism of cancer is different. It's the reason that PET scans work. They're advanced scans that pick up high levels of glucose (sugar) metabolism, thus pinpointing with great accuracy the location of tumour activity in the body. Despite this, until recently, few people had any time for the idea that this metabolic uniqueness might be useful for treatment. So again, I was frustrated by the obvious void in the information available.

That's why this book is so important to me. I want to give women in their middle years a place to find a story that resonates, that answers so many of the questions I had—that I'm sure you'll have too. I want to use my background as a Registered Dietitian and all-around health nerd to share what I know about the new-but-old field of cancer metabolism. My path in the last few years has taken me back into private practice as a low-carb dietitian and health coach. I'm a pretty good adult educator and a comfortable public speaker. As a dear friend said to me when I told her about my cancer diagnosis, "It's almost as though everything in your life so far has steered you to this point, ready to go forward as the Keto Cancer Dietitian."

I hope this book will find its way into the hands of women living with ovarian cancer and provide hope and empowerment to thrive during that journey. It's partly my own story and partly a how-to book. But it's much bigger than that. All cancers have a damaged metabolism and can be impacted by the nutritional interventions discussed in this book (1). All people with cancer can use the mental, emotional, and spiritual strategies that helped me travel through this new landscape called cancer.

You don't need a degree in biology or psychology to understand this information or to use it. Maybe you're at the very beginning of your journey, still reeling from a diagnosis, or you might be making decisions regarding treatment strategies. Whatever stage you are at, there are actionable steps in this book that you can use every day of your cancer experience and long into the future as well. With current cancer treatments and these foundational health strategies, you will have a long and awesome life ahead. This is my wish for you, dear reader.

Part 1
My Story

The Fateful Plank

It couldn't be me…I'm so healthy!

Healthy was practically my middle name—certainly a big part of my personal and professional identity. I'm a Registered Dietitian—isn't eating well for best health what I do? Well, yes, actually, it's exactly what I was doing, at least most of the time.

I was 58 years old, at an optimal weight, fully engaged in a whole range of activities—professional, personal, spiritual, and physical. It was high summer and I'd just started running again, something that makes me so very happy. Running, at least my definition of it, means shuffling up the beautiful county roads and nature trails around my home in rural Grey County, within sight of the glistening waters of Georgian Bay. At that pace, I can complete 8 km (5 miles) in about an hour at a walk/run. I love running long and slow. I've been doing it since I was 40, completing two walking marathons (42 km), then countless running half marathons over the next 15 years or so. My goal has always been to simply enjoy the experience and reap the health benefits that come from the activity.

If I had the choice, I'd skip bodyweight exercises altogether. I did them sporadically, but I certainly didn't love them. But thanks to a text from a friend of mine reminding me that I said I'd do planks, I discovered a cyst.

"So what are you up to on your plank?"

Laura is one of my oldest and dearest friends. We've been friends since Grade 7, over 40 years. She's one of my "Cottage Girls," the foursome of high school friends and "sisters-from-other-mothers" that I consider the most important female connections in my life. A recently retired elementary school teacher, she'd been training in a gym over the winter with a specific and very ambitious fitness goal— – to have the physical strength to be a "monkey" at the motorcycle racetrack. This involves being a side-car-clinging counterbalance rider in a careening motorcycle on a curvy racetrack, literally holding on for dear life. So as part of her training, she was going for a two-minute plank—see? Ambitious! At our biannual reunion in late May, I'd been inspired by her dedication and decided to recommit to doing my own bodyweight exercises, hence the follow-up text.

Well…I had no idea what my "plank was up to," as I hadn't done one in over a month. I was running but not much else. I got up from the couch and proceeded to lie down on my living room floor, readying myself for a plank.

You start by lying prone on your belly, then lift yourself up onto your toes and elbows, using all your core muscles to maintain your body in a straight horizontal line for as long as possible. Despite no movement, it's darn hard and within a few seconds, your abdominal, hip, leg, and arm muscles are all quivering and you're breathing heavily with the exertion of maintaining that difficult position against gravity. A 90-second plank is considered mastery by fitness trainers. Laura was going for 120 seconds. I would be lucky to manage 45…

Now, I never, ever, lie flat on my belly. I don't sleep on my stomach—hurts my neck to even be that way for a short while. I can do it for a massage, with a proper table to keep my neck aligned, but never otherwise. I have no grandchildren or nearby grand-puppy pets that would encourage me to lie down so completely prone on the floor. It just doesn't happen in my world.

As soon as I lowered my belly onto the carpeted floor of my living room, I knew something was wrong. It felt like I was lying on an egg in my lower belly. A solid-feeling lump—ominous…as I slid my hand in between the floor and my tummy to palpate the shape, my mind was already sounding alarms. What could this be? How could I have not noticed it before? Think, think, think…that's what a rational, pragmatic, left-brainer does, right? No wild flights of fancy into doom and gloom, but an immediate start down the path of rational explanation. Must deal with this, must figure this out…

So I sat back up, reached for the phone and called my doctor to make an appointment. It turned out to be for five days later, soonest I could get in. When my husband, Mike, came back in the house from wherever he'd been, I immediately told him what I'd found. This was no time for secrecy or trying to pretend that something major hadn't just changed in our world. There was something there, no question, and it had to be addressed.

Mike and I have been together for over 40 years. We met while working at a residential camp for disabled children in the late seventies, then long-distance dated for seven years and have been married for 33 years. We're a good team, similar in our mindsets, always having each other's backs. Although our interests and passions go in different directions, we support each other's activities.

And we're both pragmatists. So the news of the lump wasn't greeted with any sort of panic. Mike's response was, "Let's see what the doc says." Mine was to head to Google and start trying to figure it out for myself. By the time I saw my doctor the following week, I'd decided that I likely had a uterine fibroid, big enough that it was going to have to come out.

Unfortunately, that's not what my doctor thought…she palpated my lower belly with a concerned expression and several nondescript but definitely not encouraging noises. With her more experienced hands, she could feel not only the shape but also the texture of the mass in my belly. Step one, she said, was an urgent ultrasound.

The "urgent" ultrasound was booked for another five days hence, on the morning of August 1. By that afternoon, my doctor had delivered the news that I had a "huge" ovarian cyst. A simple, fluid-filled cyst but enormous nonetheless. She used the word "huge" three times in that conversation. My cyst measured 15–16 cm. The largest she'd previously seen, in 21 years of practice, was about 8 cm. Okay, that's big.

She assured me that, since it was a simple fluid cyst with no complicating features, the chances of it being cancer were very small. Still, I'd been right about one thing when making my self-diagnosis: it *was* going to have to come out.

And so began my journey.

Family History – What Made Me Who I Am

"I will love the light for it shows me the way, yet I will endure the darkness for it shows me the stars."
— **Og Mandino**

One of the first things you get asked when screening for cancer or dealing with cancer is whether you have a family history of cancer. Well, yes, as a matter of fact, I *do* have a family history of cancer. But let me explain why this was never a concern for me:

My mother had premenopausal breast cancer, diagnosed when she was 45. She died at age 55 of metastatic cancer. That statement seems pretty straightforward, but let me tell you about my amazing mother before you jump to any conclusions about her and her cancer.

My mother, Marie, was the oldest child of a farming family that lived just outside Wiarton, Ontario, on the Bruce Peninsula. She grew up working on the farm, attending public school in the local village, and playing with her many cousins, who lived in the close-knit community. Her family were devout churchgoers with a strong faith. By the age of seven, she had a younger sister, Helen, and a younger brother, Carl. That's when she contracted poliomyelitis, a life-threatening viral infection. Polio, which was also known as infantile paralysis, could cause paralysis and muscle wasting of both voluntary muscles, like legs, and involuntary muscles, such as those used to breathe. In the early twentieth century, children whose involuntary muscles were affected often died or ended up in a machine called an Iron Lung, which applied external pressure to the patient's body to make the chest cavity expand and contract to pull oxygen into the lungs: "Breathing." It was a precarious and awful existence, one spent completely immobilized, horizontally, with only the poor child's head sticking out of this steel monstrosity. They were totally cared for by staff, with nothing to occupy their minds. I can't imagine…

My mother's disease affected her legs and torso rather than her lungs, leaving her with a withered and limp lower left leg that didn't grow at the same speed as its partner. Mom limped badly, and as she grew, her spine became quite disfigured by the disparity in leg length and resulting muscle weakness in her core. She developed a marked kyphosis, with her ribs sticking out at strange angles and her spine twisted to one side. Despite being large-boned and once destined to be 5'7" or taller, she never grew past 4'11." If she'd been the child of an educated urban couple, she might have received more interventions to prevent these physical deformities but she wasn't. What she did receive from her family was a strong faith, an indomitable spirit, and an incredible capacity for love.

All of this took place during the Great Depression. Mom got polio in 1931, a hard time for the whole nation. The toll that a sick child and a hurting society took on my grandparents is almost unimaginable. But Mom recovered enough to return to school and she completed elementary school in her nearby village, then high school in Wiarton. My Aunt Helen tells of how she had to drive the horse and cutter the three miles into Wiarton every day in the winter so my mom could attend school, since she couldn't walk that far in the snow. But she graduated and set a course for herself that would result in amazing independence.

Mom attended a secretarial college in Owen Sound and then applied for a job with the Civil Service office pool in Ottawa. For this diminutive, markedly disabled young woman, travelling across the province to take up residence and a new career in the nation's capital was quite an accomplishment. She had a job in the office pool, taught a Sunday School class at the Ottawa congregation that she attended, and took a vacation to Florida with some friends. Pictures taken on her trips home show a well-dressed and very independent looking young woman with a brilliant smile and permed hair. She may not have thought that a "normal" life of marriage, babies, and housework was in her future, and for quite a while it wasn't, but at age 32 or so, something wonderful happened. Her friend Ruth took her to a party and introduced her to her boyfriend's buddy, Tom. The rest, as they say, is history.

Tom was also a "late bloomer" on the dating scene. He, too, was markedly shorter than the average guy. Maybe that was the start of the attraction—I'll never know—but they dated, married, and started a family. For someone with Mom's challenges, this was a big deal. For one thing, there wasn't much room in her abdomen for a pregnancy. Caring for boisterous babies must have taken all her energy, yet she had two children in two years, not wasting any time since she was already 36 when I was born and 38 when my brother, Peter, came along. Eventually, we added a cat and a dog to the mix as well. Mom was a full-time housewife, plus a church school and girls' club leader. Added to that, every month she typed the district newsletter for the church, printed over 300 copies on a giant hand-cranked Gestetner machine in our dining room, then hand collated, stapled, labelled, and mailed them all to the Northern Ontario congregations. As kids, of course, we were all pressed into service to help with this big undertaking. In the days before computers, all the labels were typed out by hand on her big old black typewriter. Every…month…

In 1969, when I was nine and she was 45, she was diagnosed with breast cancer. I remember little of that time, probably because my parents protected me from most of the drama. I know that Mom had a radical mastectomy, a vicious surgery that left her with a scar from her navel to deep into her armpit. As far as I know, there was no follow-up treatment. Chemo didn't exist back then and radiation wasn't available in our mid-sized Northern Ontario community. So she recovered and life went on, with school, church, after-school activities, and travel throughout Southern Ontario several times per year to visit the grandparents and extended family. It was a wonderful time.

Somewhere in my early high school days, Mom started getting pain in her hips. Given her deformities, this wouldn't have been unusual. She was diagnosed with arthritis and given meds. Not much relief. Then she was told she had bursitis, an inflammatory flare-up in her hip joint, and was prescribed cortisone shots. She decided not to do them. Finally, Aunt Helen, by then a nurse at a big teaching hospital in London, got her an appointment with a doctor there who diagnosed her with metastatic bone cancer in her spine and hips. London was about eight hours' drive from where we were living but Mom spent most of one summer being treated at Victoria Hospital with a new technology called Cobalt treatments. She returned home after this time and there followed two years or so of reasonable health, but the cancer returned and she again spent a summer in London having high-dose radiation, which made her feel very unwell. Dad and Peter and I would do the long drives to London to visit. Finally, she was able to come home but she was not cured. Her condition continued to fail gradually and in November of that year she was hospitalized again, this time in North Bay, suddenly unable to use her lower extremities. She never came home again.

Luckily, we lived about six blocks from that hospital. I was in Grade 13 at the time, already dating Mike, although he lived four hours away in Toronto and we only saw each other every few weeks. My days consisted of school, homework, trying to reach Mike by archaic long-distance phone calls, writing him anguished letters of love (by snail mail), and visiting Mom in the hospital every day. I was also the main cook at home and support to Dad. A role like that matures one quickly.

Mom died in the hospital on March 3, 1979. I was 18. We had had time to prepare for her death but nothing really prepares one for the actual loss and emptiness that follows a period of palliation like that. It was the end of second term; time to write exams for my Grade 13 courses and decide my future path. I don't really remember how I got through that period, but I do remember having little interest in a long, drawn-out, post-secondary education. I know that my friends, those same ones that are now my "Cottage Girls," were there for me throughout that year. Mike, despite being so far away and with nothing like today's communication at our disposal, was also a bedrock of support.

Somehow, we stumbled through that period as a family and came out the other side. A big part of it was the way in which my mother had looked at her world through those months and years of her illness. She was blessed with almost 10 years after her first diagnosis in which to watch and support her kids, be an example of positivity and joy, sharing, and generosity—not just for us but for many others as well—in our community, in our church family, and likely in the hospital during those long winter months of her decline. I know that much of my inner strength, resilience, and positive outlook are a legacy of my mother and her journey through her often-challenging life. I am blessed to be who I am because of her.

Mom was an outlier when it came to cancer. She was the only one in a large and extended family to develop breast cancer, or any cancer, for that matter. Her own mother and aunt both lived into their mid-nineties in robust good health. Her two sisters continue to be healthy, one at 93 and the other in her mid-eighties. Her female cousin, with whom she shared double genetics (two sisters married two brothers) also lived into her nineties. Of that woman's seven (yes—seven!) daughters, only one has developed cancer. Pretty good odds…

Given my mom's health history, I always believed I didn't have a genetic predisposition to getting a hormonal cancer but that something in Mom's environment had likely made her more susceptible. Who knows what she was given or what was done to her during her long journey with polio and its aftereffects? We know that Mom spent one summer in a body cast in a hospital in Toronto after back surgery. In the 1930s and '40s, did we really know what we were giving to patients? Especially young women on the edge of puberty?

Aside from her remote health history, Mom wasn't able to do many of the things that we consider protective against the development of cancer. She was never overweight but she couldn't be physically active, a known risk reducer. Having your babies before age 30 and breastfeeding them are considered to reduce risk but Mom did neither of these things. Breastfeeding was discouraged, especially for a "special" mom like her. Having bottles that Dad could be responsible for was likely a godsend for her. Her diet would have been basic and clean, typical of the diets of the 1960s: Meat, potatoes, vegetables (often frozen or canned), brown bread, peanut butter, canned fruit for dessert. Little eating out. No alcohol whatsoever. A big treat was an occasional bag of potato chips brought home from the store and divided into four bowls. Likewise, soft drinks like Coca-Cola were brought home occasionally, with the bottle being divided into four single glasses. Canada Dry Ginger Ale was only for when you were sick—I can't drink it to this day because of that association…

So, yes, there's cancer in my immediate family history. But do I think that that has anything to do with my current cancer? No. Do I think that it affects my current outlook on life and my own journey with cancer? You bet! I have this amazing life example of the woman that was my mother—

strong, joyful, resilient, faithful, loving, generous, and positive. Although she's been gone for almost 40 years, well over half my life, I know that I am who I am because of her influence. For that, I feel so very blessed and eternally grateful.

The Doctor Parade

Summer is short and precious to Canadians. In the span of roughly nine weeks, everyone in the whole country wants to take at least two weeks' vacation: Kids are out of school, nights are short, and days are long and warm. In the world of business, lots of things get put on hold over the summer months. As a health practitioner, I've noticed that the various conferences and other events of a professional life are all clustered into a few months in spring and again in fall, with winter considered too dicey for scheduling because of the weather, while summer is left open for vacations. I live in vacation/cottage country, so I'm very aware of the fact that the entire summer is compressed into just 10 weeks. By mid-June, things are ramping up in the tourist villages and on local beaches. During July and August, you can hardly move for the influx of city visitors, and then in September, on the Tuesday after Labour Day weekend, suddenly everything is deserted. Not because the weather is any different than it was the week before—just that "summer" has been declared over. Schools resume classes, all extra activities start up again, and we go into our "fall" mindset: "Well, that was a great summer…now let's ramp our lives back up to their regular full throttle."

So finding out that I had a large ovarian cyst at the beginning of August was not great timing. A 2013 study has shown that, in summer, longer wait times for specialist doctor appointments have actually been measured—it's a real issue (2).

Despite the assurances of my family doctor that my cyst was very unlikely to be cancer, I was anxious to get moving on getting the thing out.

Of course, being who I am—a medical nerd and lifelong learner—I had taken a headfirst dive into the internet for information about ovarian cysts. Blogs, articles, research, videos…I watched laparoscopic cyst removal surgery several times on YouTube. People would get all squidgy when I would tell them about it, but for me, it seemed like the obvious thing to do.

The day of the initial diagnosis, I'd been read the riot act about risky activities that could cause the cyst to rupture. Even small cysts (1 cm or more) can cause excruciating pain if they rupture. The first restriction was that I shouldn't be running. I finally get all the physical issues from a stress fracture behind me, get my mind and motivation in the right place, have worked myself up to doing 5-milers several days a week, and now you tell me I have to stop cold turkey? I was pissed.

Other restrictions included anything that placed me at risk of a fall or sudden jolt. No jumping off things and landing hard. Even plopping myself down into a chair, the kind of thing that I tend to do when tired, was a potential source of sudden pain. No exercises that placed excessive internal pressure on my core, such as the plank or lifting heavy weights. And none of the "bump and grind" aspects of sexual relations with my husband. Well, that one stung!

My "urgent" referral to our local gynecology team resulted in a three-week wait for a first consult with a locum doctor. The doctor who had received my referral was away on a month's leave so I met with her replacement, a lovely young woman from London, in mid-August. She examined me, looked at the ultrasound results and agreed that the cyst would have to come out. We discussed surgical options—laparoscopic surgery vs. open surgery—and what that would look like. She agreed that there appeared to be little chance that the cyst was cancerous, given its apparently simple structure. However, since she was just the fill-in doc, I would still need to be seen by the actual surgeon and booked into her surgery schedule. She was back at work the second week of September and had her first surgery date on September 28—a full six weeks away! But that date was already full so I would have to wait for an appointment on October 10—almost eight weeks away! So much for "urgent."

During this time, the cyst continued to grow and cause more symptoms. I never had acute pain unless I did something stupid, like the day I returned to my office in late afternoon, tired or frustrated by something (I can't remember anymore), and plopped myself back into my office chair with a thud. Sudden pain coursed through my lower abdomen causing me to catch my breath and go rigid. Holy crap! What had I just done? I was terrified that I had caused a rupture, but it turned out that it had just shifted, yanking on its connective tissues, which caused the pain. I lowered myself more carefully into chairs after that.

I had to go out and buy myself different clothes to accommodate the swelling in my abdomen, which now rose above the level of my belly button. I was wearing the same size clothes but now I was thick through the waist like I was in mid-pregnancy. Value Village became my new best shopping spot, looking for yoga pants without any tight waist elastic and loose, flowy tops that hid the thickness. Even so, when I sat down, I usually had to pull the waistband of my pants up over the top of the bulge to be comfortable. Curiously, though, during the slow parade of doctors' appointments, nobody seemed concerned that the cyst was growing this rapidly.

I met with the local gynecologist, Dr. C, in mid-September and was quite comfortable with her. We discussed the details of the surgery and she stated clearly, "If I thought that this was cancer, I would not be the one doing this surgery. I would be referring you to a gynecological oncologist in London." Mind you, everyone was still making judgements and decisions based on the first and only ultrasound, taken six weeks earlier. We decided that if the second ovary (which they hadn't even been able to see on the original ultrasound) was intact, that they would leave it in place. I was hoping that this might help to maintain my flagging hormones as I was well past menopause. I am of the firm belief that everything inside of us is there for a reason so why remove more than is necessary? The doctor agreed but said that if they found a cyst on the second ovary, both would come out. My fallopian tubes were also to be removed. She warned me that there was always the chance that I might wake up to a full abdominal incision and more missing parts, depending on what she found. But all things considered, I was still very much of the mindset that I was just dealing with a big old fluid-filled cyst, nothing more than a random nuisance.

Luckily, in the end, I was offered a cancellation spot on the doctor's first available surgery, on September 28. Being a Friday, and right at the end of the month, it was absolutely the most convenient timing for my business responsibilities. I booked two weeks off from my nursing homes, moved around my few private clients, and prepared to be slow for a few days. On the morning of surgery, while fasting, I prepared a pot of my favourite curried squash soup and defrosted some low-carb bread, ready for a comfort food supper when I got home. I was ready to go.

The Big C — Life Invasion, or Is That Inversion?

"Be not a slave of your own past —
plunge into the sublime seas, dive deep, and swim far,
so you shall come back with new self-respect,
with new power, and with an advanced experience
that shall explain and overlook the old."

— Ralph Waldo Emerson

Day surgery is a wonderful thing. Being able to sleep in your own bed the night before (though I expect most people don't sleep much, or very well) and do any preparatory work at home, then just walk into the hospital a few hours ahead of surgery time leaves people feeling more in charge of their own situation. I mean, if you must spend hours and multiple trips to the loo for bowel surgery prep, wouldn't you rather do that in your own bathroom? Or if you're fasting, wouldn't you rather have access to your own refrigerator for clear fluids, your own kettle and tea bags? I certainly would.

I was due to arrive at 10:00 a.m. for scheduled surgery at noon. Because Mike was working, a neighbour drove me in on his way to the hardware store. I had accepted a cancellation spot so although it worked for me the date was very inconvenient for our family, given that Mike was scheduled to work, then had an onstage performance in the evening at our local little theatre. But I knew all of this going in so I'd arranged for assistance from my circle of friends.

I'm fiercely independent and didn't need a family member to sit with me or wait around for me during the surgery. Hospitals, especially this one where I used to work, are familiar turf and the medical system doesn't scare me. And because my mom wasn't able to fuss over me as I was growing up, I don't take well to being fussed over. In fact, it gives me the heebie-jeebies to have someone want to "mother/smother" me.

The process of going from a person to a patient is an interesting one. It starts when you're handed a stack of hospital garb and are requested to give up every single bit of your individuality. In other words, all of your clothing, jewelry, make-up, possessions. The only things I could keep that marked me as me were my tattoos…it's a disorienting process. Then you're sent to sit in a common waiting room with a variety of other similarly de-personalized folks—all ages and genders. Some are obviously very nervous, sitting rigidly still and focussed inwardly. Some are holding hands with spouses or parents. Nobody looks relaxed or upbeat. It's a quietly anxious room.

Day surgery patients in our local hospital walk into the operating room (OR) on their own two feet. No stretchers. That's nice—it feels like, in a small way, you're still master of your own fate. But it's like walking onto the deck of a spaceship—a totally foreign place for all but those who work there. Luckily for me, there in the OR hallway was a nurse who I have known for decades, since my days of working in the hospital. A familiar face and a cozy, catching-up-on-life chat passed the time until I was called into the OR.

The surgery itself was unremarkable, except for the size of the cyst and the amount of fluid drained out of me. When Dr. C was done, she left me a handwritten note on the bottom of my discharge instructions. It said, "Martha, went great, 1,500 cc of cyst fluid!! The second cyst was on the other ovary (6–7 cm) so BOTH were removed. No more cysts, and pelvis looks really healthy. Come and see me in 4–6 weeks to review."

The anesthesiologist came by to see me in the recovery room and patted my shoulder, saying, "One and a half litres of fluid!" Like I had broken some kind of record and he was really impressed.

By 4:00 p.m., I was ready to be discharged. With some pain meds on board, I very slowly, and in considerable discomfort, got dressed and was wheeled down to the main lobby where my dear friends, Bonita and Frank, who had come to give me a ride home, were waiting for me. I was actually ahead of schedule, since I'd been sent into surgery a bit earlier than planned and, I guess, because I recovered well, so when they got me home, Mike was still there, which was comforting and reassuring for us both. Walking was uncomfortable, sitting was a little better, but the transition from upright to sitting was really painful. And lying down was almost impossibly excruciating. The closer I'd get to horizontal, the worse the pain would get, stopping me in mid-lower. Stuck in mid-air, literally, gasping with the stabbing pains.

Laparoscopic surgery doesn't leave much of an impression on the skin but the amount of stuff that is cut, burned, rearranged, and stitched inside of the abdomen is extensive and it's really sore. I had two tiny incisions, each about 1 cm (½ inch) across on my upper and mid abdomen, and one larger one, about 3 cm (1½ inch) in length down towards my groin on the left side. The highest incision had been for the camera scope, placed that high because of the size of the cyst. The other two were for the tool scopes and the largest lower incision was the exit port for all of my body parts, including the deflated cysts. I thought it was pretty impressive that something the size of a bag of milk, holding well over a litre of fluid, could be removed through a 1½-inch hole.

I got a lot of knitting done that first few days after surgery. Friends in the neighbourhood arrived with wonderful food—meat pies, casseroles, homemade granola. I entertained several friends for tea visits during that week of convalescence. In fact, I was having a visit from my cousin, Donna, on the sixth day after surgery when my cell phone rang and the caller ID said Dr. C's office.

"Hi, Martha. This is _____ from Dr. C's office. Your path report has come back."

Me: "My Pap? They did a Pap while they were in there?"

"No. Your *pathology* report. The doctor would like you to come in. She can see you tomorrow morning at 9:45. Please bring another pair of ears."

Me: "Oh, shit. That's doesn't sound good."

I was totally broadsided. I'd been assured by both my family doctor and the surgeon that my cyst was not cancerous. The process of getting it addressed and removed had taken a leisurely two and a half months. Only one ultrasound had been done, back in early August, with no follow-up screening deemed necessary, despite significant growth in the intervening two months.

Mike wandered back into the house from outside and I put on a fake smile and said that everything was fine. Donna took one look at my face and said, "Well, I'll be going now. Thanks for tea." She's a very wise woman. As soon as she left, with big hugs and whispered offers of support in any way she could help, I told Mike about the phone call. He immediately got the full implications and assumed the same "deer in the headlights" expression. Our world had just changed forever.

My No Longer Pristine Belly

Let a teacher wave away the flies and put a plaster on the wound.
Don't turn your head. Keep looking at the bandaged place.
That's where the light enters you.
And don't believe for a moment that you're healing yourself.

— Rumi, thirteenth century poet and Sufi mystic

I have no scars. Nada. I have tattoos—several—but as an adult, I have never required any significant surgery. Two babies, no stitches. One wisdom tooth extraction with a couple of stitches. And about 15 years ago, a minor procedure to remove a little hematoma from beside my eye, resulting in tiny, cosmetic surgery type stitches in the fold of my eyelid. That's it. Not a bad track record for 58 years…

After my laparoscopic surgery, I had two wee incisions that hadn't even required stitches. I think that they were simply glued together. The larger lower incision had a running stitch closure. Instead of individual stitches with spiky little ends sticking up to get caught in clothing, this incision looked like one long suture thread had been pulled through one end, woven back and forth down the incision, and then tied off at the other end. Sort of like a shoelace pulled very tightly to close the gap completely. Only one knot. Very neat. They were even self-dissolving sutures so I had no need to go anywhere to get them removed.

Despite the rather insignificant look of these incisions, however, I was assured by my medical friends that there was much more to healing than just the surface level stuff. And the amount of discomfort that I was in was

proof they were right. With laparoscopic surgery, there's a lot of rearrange-
ment of organs, cutting and cauterization (burning to close off incisions
and to stop bleeding), tugging and pulling. It took me a good few weeks to
recover my usual ability to move around without pain. Many movements
required me to hold onto my abdomen, particularly down low, and apply
pressure to prevent pain, almost like I was holding things in place as I
moved. Having taken out 1.5 litres of space-occupying cyst meant there
was a cavity that needed to be filled and organs that had to return to their
usual spots.

Once I received the news that my cyst was cancerous, further surgery
was one of the possible options for treatment. Dr. C referred me to London Regional Cancer Centre, to a gynecological oncologist surgeon, Dr. S.
When we met with him four weeks later, he did not recommend surgery
based on my diagnosis of endometrioid adenocarcinoma stage 2/3. His
recommendation was six rounds of chemotherapy to address the fact that
the cyst had been ruptured in situ. No surgery, no radiation. Chemo could
be done in Owen Sound, my own local hospital where there was a satellite
cancer centre of the LRCC. I could also have my follow-up CAT scan
(which I had requested) in Owen Sound. I was thrilled and texted friends
and family all the way home with the good news...

Well, that euphoria lasted about six days. I received a call from Dr. S
the following Monday telling me that unbeknownst to him my pathology
had been sent off for further consultation and that my diagnosis had been
changed based on the review. Now I was considered to have high-grade
serous adenocarcinoma (HGSC), stage 1C2. This is a more common but
somewhat harder-to-treat type of tumour. Chemotherapy was still the plan
but with this change in diagnosis, surgery was back on the table for discussion.

Dr. S explained to me that serous cancer cells (remember that the tumour was gone before I knew it was there so we were chasing individual
cancer cells that had escaped from the rupturing of the cyst) were "sticky,"
meaning that they liked to hang out in the abdominal cavity, seeding new
tumours on other internal organs, the walls of the abdominal cavity, the
viscera (the network of tissues that holds all of the internal organs in place),
or the omentum (the fatty structure that tends to sit in front of your internal organs). You have lots of nooks and crannies in your abdomen where

these individual cancer cells can get themselves into trouble. So now I was being offered an alternative chemo-administration pathway called intra-peritoneal (IP) administration. This would place one of the chemo meds directly into my abdominal cavity, swishing it around all those nooks and crannies. However, to do this I would have to undergo surgery to place a chemo port that drained into my abdomen, involving two incisions—one up under my ribs and a second one vertically under my navel.

For this treatment, I had to go to the London Regional Cancer Centre, some three hours away from home in the middle of the Ontario winter. It meant giving up the comfort of being treated at my local hospital, where I had previously worked and knew many people. It meant giving up being part of that local community of support.

It was a hard decision to make but I wanted to achieve the best out-come. I was determined to only do this once so decided that peritoneal chemo was the best way to go. Also, my faith in the local hospital had been shaken by wrong diagnoses several times in this process to date so it felt right to take my business to the larger clinic in London.

Once I was settled on going for the IP chemo and the resultant surgery, the next decision was whether to complete the "standard of care" for ovar-ian cancer and have a full hysterectomy while I was there. This turned out to be very hard for me. I have always believed that we were created with all our parts in place for a reason and we shouldn't take them out for no good reason. There was no proof that my uterus was involved in anything so far. It appeared pristine. On the other hand, I was long since done with it. It took several weeks of agonizing and another visit with Dr. S in London be-fore I was finally able to agree to the full abdominal hysterectomy in addi-tion to the port placement. It would mean a four-day stay in London Hos-pital and a 6-inch vertical abdominal scar. Plus, the additional two-inch scar under my breast for the port placement. In two months, I went from having a pristine belly to one with five incision scars. I felt unattractive.

Down the Rabbit Hole

I am a self-confessed health nerd. I have always been the logical, problem-solving, analytical type. Even my creative hobbies—quilting, knitting, sewing, and cooking—are pattern-based. I get panicked if I'm presented with a totally blank piece of paper and asked to create from scratch. On the other hand, patterns, puzzles, chemistry, or math problems, anything with a logical progression are endlessly attractive to me.

When I started looking into nutritional and metabolic aspects of cancer, I approached the task like a puzzle. Of course, I started where everyone does—Dr. Google.

First up was ovarian cancer itself. I wanted to know everything there was to know about *my* particular type of cancer. At first, I was given the diagnosis of "endometrioid carcinoma stage 1/2" so that's where I went. I learned about the several types of ovarian cancer—serous, endometrioid, germ cell, stromal, clear cell—30 types in all! Holy cow! Then I investigated how cancers were staged: Stage 1, 2, 3, and 4. Then within those classes, there were subclasses A, B, and C.

Once my diagnosis was changed to "high-grade serous adenocarcinoma stage 1C," I dove further down the rabbit hole searching for details of that particular cancer type and its treatments and prognosis.

As a Registered Dietitian, I'm expected to practice dietetics in an "evidence-based" way, so I've been able to find and read scientific research articles since my university days. And thanks to Google Scholar and PubMed, most anything that's been published in a scientific journal is available online. And most of it is free.

I was also able to research the specific medications that I'd be taking, their mechanism of action, their usual prescribing regimen, and their side effects and risks. Besides the scientific stuff, I watched YouTube videos of various women who were taking these drugs and their stories. Some of those videos were recorded as they lay in bed, wiped out by chemo and its side effects.

As I delved into this warren of information, it dawned on me that there was very little mentioned anywhere about how and what these women ate or drank. Almost as if nutrition wasn't significant. But gradually I became aware of a scientific undercurrent of information about the fact that cancer had its own unique metabolism and that there were possible nutritional interventions that could impact on it.

The fact that cancer is a greedy hog when it comes to glucose uptake from the blood and its exaggerated rate of metabolism has been known for a long time (3). It's how PET scans work. A PET scan is a functional test that seeks out and finds areas of hypermetabolism, areas that are sucking up and using glucose like crazy.

At the time, I wondered why nobody connected the dots between dietary sugar intake and the glucose-gluttonous cancer cells. If we knew that cancer cells use glucose (sugar) at a high rate, why hadn't it occurred to anybody that maybe having extra sugar in the bloodstream was a bad thing?

It turns out that someone had, as far back as the 1920s, but that information was lost for decades after the Second World War. It's been reintroduced in the last 20 years by several maverick researchers and scientists, but they're fighting an uphill battle to get this area of cancer research funded or investigated. There's no money to be made in telling people to eat less sugar (especially given the deep pockets and powerful lobbying interests of Big Agriculture and Big Food) and certainly no money to be made in pharmaceuticals using this approach. Much of academic research is funded by large industrial organizations with a vested interest in promoting their products or point of view. It can lead to biased studies, reporting on results that benefit their benefactors but neglecting to study areas that have no potential for financial returns. Big Industry is not interested in having their profitable medications or inexpensively produced food products made obsolete or proven unnecessary (4).

The research into cancer metabolism is currently in its infancy but is compelling in what it has revealed so far. Researchers have looked deep into cancer cells to reveal damaged micro-organelles, changes to cell membrane receptors and sensors, genetic and nuclear changes, and unusual chemical signalling. Studies on single-cell organisms and rodents (mice and rats) have been carried out with various nutritional manipulations to look at the impact on implanted human cancers. And studies on humans are underway, starting with case study reports, and progressing to interventional studies (considered the gold standard of evidence). This is an excruciatingly slow process, requiring years of grant proposals, ethics committee clearances, study design, recruitment, data collection, and then finally assessment and conclusions. All that before publication in a peer-reviewed journal to allow the information to be shared with the wider world.

For an open-minded, low-carb-leaning dietitian, this was fascinating information. I have summarized what I found in the chapters, Cancer is a Metabolic Disease and What This Means for Cancer Treatment in Part 2 of this book. Once I found this area of research, I consumed everything I could find from researchers like Thomas Seyfried, Miriam Kalamian, Dom D'Agostino, and Valter Longo. I bought books, watched lectures, downloaded and read scientific articles, and listened to podcasts and audiobooks. It became a bit of an obsession.

It boggled my mind that almost nobody had really connected this information together with people's actual dietary intake. Dietitians and the cancer institutes and associations around the world were still telling everyone the same thing. Eat whatever stays down; focus on getting enough calories for prevention of weight loss. Use commercial nutritional products such as Ensure and Boost to supplement your intake. All highly processed and full of industrial seed oils and sugars—yuck. Eat small and often. Suck on candies. Sip on ginger ale. Every single recommendation was based on sugar or industrial, genetically modified, conventionally raised (meaning chemical-laden) seed oils. Every recommendation was something that would drive up blood sugars and insulin levels in the blood —exactly what cancer cells need to thrive.

What the heck were we doing?

Even my preoperative instructions mentioned eating or drinking lots of high-carbohydrate foods and beverages prior to surgery (up until the fasting period of a few hours preop) and then bringing your own nutritional supplements (Ensure was recommended) to the hospital for the immediate postop period. Yeah, I ignored that part.

I did go to the local drug store and find some low-carb canned meal replacements, meant to be for post-gym workouts, I guess. It was like a chocolate SlimFast drink in a can. I dutifully took them to the hospital with me. I drank one of them the day after surgery—bad idea. Within an hour, I was nauseous and vomited the whole thing back up. My only post-surgical complication and it was self-inflicted. I gave the remaining cans to one of my nurses, who expressed an interest in them, and went back to eating hard-boiled eggs and cheese packets.

Maybe I shouldn't have been surprised to find that eating the foods that made me feel good in healthy times would also help my body through harder times. Who knew that nutrition, the very thing that I had been studying and practicing as a career my whole life, could be so powerful? Even if I hadn't realized it, however, it turned out at least a few people had…

The work of PhD researcher Valter Longo, in particular, was focussed on fasting and its role in impacting chemotherapy (5). His work proved that fasting didn't negatively impact on the effectiveness of the chemo medications and that, in fact, it appeared to be a factor in making chemo more effective by placing stress on the cancer cells. His lab at the University of California, Los Angeles, also published several articles—based on experiments using organisms ranging from single-celled yeast, to mice, to humans—showing that chemo remained effective on cancer cells even as fasting protected healthy cells, therefore resulting in fewer side effects. His seminal paper on these findings was a case study series of 10 human patients who fasted through some or all of their chemo treatments and reported on their side effects and quality-of-life markers (6). Almost uniformly, the fasted chemo sessions were better tolerated.

This idea was further developed by Dr. Thomas Seyfried, a researcher at Boston College Department of Biology, in what he calls his Press/Pulse theory (7). He proposes that cancer cells can be "pressed" or stressed by keeping blood sugars, circulating insulin, and insulin-like growth factors low, thus depriving them of what they need for unregulated growth. Once in this sorry state, any treatment that's meant to attack the cells—chemotherapy, radiation therapy, hyperbaric oxygen, high dose IV vitamin C, or other newer drug therapies—will be much more effective in destroying the tumour cells. He has extensive mouse data to support these interventions and several human case studies. It is worth noting that most of his work so far has been on brain cancers (8).

The idea underlying all this is that nutritional interventions that cause your body to be more inhospitable to cancer cells (with their disordered metabolism and heavy glucose requirements) and protective of your healthy cells (normal metabolism) can be combined with traditional or newer therapies to deliver a one-two punch to cancer. Fasting, a ketogenic diet, or a combination of both won't cure cancer on their own but they do set the stage for better response to conventional therapies. It's the secret superpower that boosts the effectiveness of traditional approaches.

How I Became a Renegade Low-Carb Dietitian

Dietitians are not known to be very open-minded when it comes to low-carb diets. We are proud members of the traditional medical establishment and tend to cling tenaciously to the idea that we are the nutrition experts and should be the only credible resource persons in that intellectual space. This is a rather elitist position and has left RDs open to criticism from many other non-RD experts that we are blinkered and closed-minded. For the most part, they're right.

I had an interest in health and nutrition since my high school days and though I originally thought about physiotherapy, when it came to choosing a path, nutrition won out. I attended a four-year university program and a one-year hospital-based internship and proudly accepted my RD pin at the end of that time.

My university years, 1980–84, coincided perfectly with the 1980 Nutrition Guidelines for Americans, the first ever nutrition guidelines that made recommendations to all Americans to eat a low-fat diet. The report was the brainchild of a large commission in the US called the McGovern Commission. Senator McGovern and his coinvestigators were heavily lobbied and influenced by the work of a researcher named Ancel Keys and the American Heart Association. There was also great pressure from the industrial agricultural complex in the US, which produced vast quantities of monocrop commodities such as corn, soybeans, and wheat. Despite an almost complete absence of rigorous scientific studies to support their position, they released low-fat guidelines that then went on to influence the national nutrition guidelines of all Western countries.

The low-fat dietary paradigm was considered cutting-edge science when I was training and all the textbooks and practice manuals were duly revised to reflect this new way of thinking. Saturated fat was a killer, cholesterol caused coronary plaques and heart attacks, and meat should be strictly rationed. Full-fat dairy products, especially butter, were dangerously full of both cholesterol and saturated fats—oh horrors! And eggs? Absolutely evil!

I practiced as an RD using these underlying beliefs and guidelines for the first 22 years of my career. Whether in hospital, working in homecare, private practice, or as a long-term care consultant dietitian, I can honestly say that I was of minimal help to my patients and clients, but we all had to toe the party line regarding what was deemed to be a "healthy" diet. We dietitians were famously critical—and dismissive—of Dr. Atkins and his low-carb diet. I happily trashed him and his approach along with my colleagues during that time.

In 2007, while browsing in a bookstore, I happened upon a little book called *The Shangri-La Diet* by the psychologist Seth Roberts. Its premise was the idea that taking flavourless calories could trick the body into appetite suppression and hence less food intake. He proposed taking shots of flavourless oils, supplying pure fat, between meals. Since I had always struggled with about 20 stubborn extra pounds that wouldn't come off no matter what I tried, I decided to give this crazy idea a go. It was my first time "thinking outside the box" on nutrition, and it exposed my mind to a whole new world of alternative nutritional perspectives and to the idea that dietitians perhaps *didn't* have the whole nutrition world locked down. And I lost weight! In hindsight, I know that the dietary pattern of the Shangri-La diet would have been impacting on my hormones, but at the time, it seemed like magic.

As I learned more about sugars and the role of carbohydrates in the body's physiology, I became more and more unsettled with promoting the status quo nutritional recommendations. How could foods that have nourished humans over millions of years of development suddenly be deadly? How could meat and animal fats be dangerous? At the same time, humans were getting fatter and sicker by the year. Obesity, Type 2 diabetes, hypertension, Alzheimer's disease, and cancers were all increasing rapidly through the end of the twentieth century and into the twenty-first. Something was wrong…

I had been eating progressively more low carb over the ensuing years and was feeling fabulous. Despite entering menopause, I was cruising through my fifties; I had boundless energy, nothing ached, I was on no medication, and the food was delicious. I wasn't strictly keto or even 100 percent low-carb, but overall, there was little sugar or grains in my diet and I ate lots of whole unprocessed foods and healthy fats.

By 2016, I couldn't sit by any longer and spout the conventional wisdom. I decided to put my money where my mouth was and get some additional training in low-carb nutrition. I signed up for the Primal Health Coach certification through Primal Blueprint and completed that course over the summer. That led me to starting up Primal RD, a private practice using a Low Carb Healthy Fats (LCHF) approach to address healthy aging and chronic disease management. Excitedly, I rented office space, created my teaching materials, set up a website, and started the promotion of my new service. This included mailings to all the family doctors in my small Ontario city, about 35 in total. I figured that at least some of them had to be seeing patients with questions about low carb and the latest "fad" diet—keto. The response was deafening silence. Second and third mailings had the same response. A request to do a "lunch and learn" talk at the health team office (where most of them were located) was denied. The conventional wisdom was clearly very strong with the doctors and the family health team dietitians. It was discouraging.

That was when cancer entered my life. I had a strong belief in the truth of the Low Carb Healthy Fats dietary approach, including its more extreme cousin, the Well Formulated Ketogenic Diet. Support for its use has been growing steadily, with evidence to back up its application in diabetes, metabolic syndrome, weight management, inflammatory diseases, mental health disorders, and dementia. Gradually, more health professionals, even dietitians, have been realizing the power of these nutritional approaches and changing their recommendations to their patients, with impressive results. A Canadian online group, Canadian Clinicians for Therapeutic Nutrition (CCTN), has been formed to bring these clinicians together—a nationwide group of doctors, pharmacists, nurses, and dietitians. This group works to support other clinicians to "come out" of the low-carb closet and promote their use of nutritional therapies without fear of recrimination. As this nutritional approach becomes more mainstream, the hope is that the feeling of being on the fringe will be lessened.

So I remain a renegade but not quite as lonely a renegade as before.

Build Your Foundation – Keto Diet Basics

This section of the book will start at the very beginning of how to implement a ketogenic diet for therapeutic benefits. A ketogenic diet is simply a pattern of eating that puts your body into a metabolic state where you are producing ketones from fat molecules (either diet-derived or bodyfat-derived) and using them for fuel in your cells. This is called "nutritional ketosis," but throughout this book, I will refer to it as simply ketosis. Ketones are small water-soluble molecules that your body uses as a fuel source. The actual foods used to do this can be quite varied or could be no foods at all (fasting is the quickest way to get into ketosis).

A keto diet can be done eating nothing but pepperoni sticks, pork rinds, and cheese, but this is not a healthy diet and doesn't benefit your body. The optimal keto diet is going to give you adequate, but not excessive, protein for maintaining your lean muscle mass, lots of minerals and nutrients to promote the best possible operation of your healthy cells, good support for your gut microbiome, and adequate fat to ensure that you are not hungry and that your meals are satiating. And as a bonus, your meals should taste delicious and make you feel supported and pampered, not restricted and undernourished.

Imagine bacon and eggs or a spinach and feta cheese omelette for breakfast. Imagine a large Caesar salad with no croutons but instead crunchy bacon pieces, rich savoury dressing, Parmesan cheese flakes throughout, and a piece of grilled chicken or salmon lying on top. Imagine a rich bowl of creamy mushroom soup, followed by a ribeye steak and grilled asparagus with olive oil and balsamic vinegar drizzled over it. Followed by a bowl of blueberries with whipping cream poured over the top. These are all keto-genic-compliant meals. And totally delicious.

The absolute crux of the keto diet is the restriction of carbohydrates to a level that forces your body to switch to a fat-burning metabolism. So our ketogenic diet will be adequate in protein, very low in carbohydrates, have enough fat for satiety, and include good sources of minerals and vitamins. It's also designed to prevent inflammatory irritation.

The Basic Rules

Stop all sugar consumption. All regular pop, candy, desserts and baked items, cookies, sweet sauces, such as BBQ sauce or ketchup in large quantities. All juices and "fruit drinks," iced tea, lemonade. Flavoured yogurt or kefir that have added sugar. All added white or brown sugar in other foods. Honey and syrups.

Get rid of all industrial seed oils in your house. No canola, corn, soy, or vegetable oils, no margarine. The diet is based on fat but it has to be healthy fat.

Try to avoid all refined grain products. That's bread, crackers, biscuits, pasta.

No matter which level of carb restriction you're aiming for, whether moderate low carb, stricter low carb or full-on ketogenic diet, the above rules apply. Actually, they should apply to everyone, every day. We'd all be healthier.

Why? Think about our ancient ancestors. They only had access to any significant amount of sugar or starchy foods in the summer and fall, when plants were ripening fruit or growing starchy roots or tubers. The only other major source of sugar was honey, a rare treat and very hard to obtain. And the reason to eat as much sugary fruits, starchy roots, and honey as possible was to fatten up for the much leaner winter season. Even in tropical areas, there were seasons of abundance and seasons of scarcity throughout the year.

The rest of our ancestors' diet was made up of animal foods that could be hunted, trapped, or gathered (think insects), plus storable plant materials, such as tubers and nuts as a backup for the days when animal foods were not available. Smoking and drying allowed for storage of meats and other animal parts when they were in abundance. And the fat of the animals was gathered and stored as a precious commodity with numerous uses besides being consumed as food.

Our ancient ancestors would have spent much of their time in mild to moderate ketosis. They needed to be able to go for significant stretches of time with minimal or no food intake, yet remain mentally sharp enough and physically powerful enough to manage to hunt and/or gather their next meal. And even after a period of starvation, once dug or gathered, many foods would have to be prepared before any calories could be consumed. Plant foods, in particular, would have required scraping, pounding, soaking, and possibly cooking before being edible, as most calorie-dense plant foods (such as tubers, roots, seeds, and nuts) need processing before they are safe for human consumption. Remember too that fruits, potatoes, berries, grains, and beans were not the big, fat, juicy, sweet, or starchy hybrid plants that we have now. They were tiny, tart, seedy, or hard—basically inedible without processing.

Animal foods, on the other hand, could be consumed fresh and raw, basically as soon as the animal was dead. The remainder would be processed by cooking, drying, smoking, or salting to provide nutrition for the future. Here's an interesting description of pemmican, the traditional storage form of meat and fat for indigenous North Americans:

Pemmican consists of lean, dried meat (beef, bison, deer, or elk) which is crushed to a powder and mixed with an equal amount of hot, rendered fat, usually beef tallow. Sometimes crushed, dried berries are added as well. For long periods of time, people can subsist entirely on pemmican, drawing on the fat for energy and the protein for strength, and liver glucose production, when needed.

Note that this food was a 50/50 mix of lean dried meat and fat. The berries, if available, were simply a bonus, for flavour. They would have supplied some additional nutrients but weren't considered essential. Even these ancestral people understood the importance of fat in satiety and nutritional adequacy.

If you haven't been following a low-carb diet prior to this, you will need to start your journey to keto by becoming more metabolically flexible, a process that is referred to as becoming "fat-adapted." This metabolic state also makes it much easier to fast. To achieve this, you will cut back on your carbohydrate intake and increase your fat intake until your body receives the signal that it needs to develop its metabolic pathways to address the new balance of energy coming in. When we consume carbs at every eating opportunity, every couple of hours, we never burn fats and so our innate fat-burning machinery is effectively mothballed and disassembled. For more information about fat burning, carb burning, and the mechanisms that impact on them, I would recommend The Obesity Code by Dr. Jason Fung. (See Books and Blogs list in Appendix 2.)

Quality Matters, but Only Kinda...

There's lots of buzz in the keto community about eating the highest quality foods. "Grass-fed, grass-finished" meats, pasture-raised poultry, free-range eggs, wild game, A2 dairy, organic vegetables, and fruits—the list goes on and on. It sounds very elitist and can make adopting healthy dietary changes sound like a difficult and expensive process.

Nothing could be further from the truth. "The best quality food that you can afford"—that's the message to listen to instead. If this way of eating relied on only the hoity-toity foods, the vast majority of people would not be able to benefit from it.

There's also the matter of access—not everyone lives in a rural area with access to farmers, farmers markets, butcher shops, or high-end organic whole food restaurants. The reality of life for many people is shopping for their groceries at Walmart, discount-style grocery stores, Costco-type stores, and even convenience stores. The concept of a "food desert," urban areas where there's no food shopping available within walking distance, is a real thing in many cities. Fixed incomes are a major impactor on food choices for the elderly, the unemployed, the disabled, and the working poor. Using public transit means no roomy car trunk for your groceries or door-to-door convenience, which means shopping "little and often."

So how do you get your "keto" on? To the best of your ability, that's how! Tune out the Facebook groups and websites that insist that only elitist foods are worthy of your health improvement journey. The keto diet is just as much about what you remove from your diet as it is about what you eat. Simply by removing the foods in the previous "The Basic Rules" list, you have already made a vast improvement in your health trajectory.

I'm all for eating the best that you can afford. I am blessed to live in a rural area where I have access to a lovely weekly farmers market with local fish, locally raised beef, lamb, pork, and chicken, and locally grown vegetables in season. I'm also friends with several of the farmers that produce this stuff and can visit their farms and buy from them directly. I have a butcher that produces local beef within an easy drive. I'm also blessed to have a car for driving there and an income from my day job as a long-term care consultant dietitian that has allowed me the luxury of buying from these places.

But much of my produce is purchased at the local No Frills and I shop the sales on basics. I cringe when paying for bags of macadamia nuts or almond flour at the local bulk store. I stock up when canned salmon or butter go on sale.

Keto doesn't require macadamia nuts, ribeye steaks, or canned salmon. It can be done well with ground beef, chicken leg quarters, and on-sale flaked tuna. You don't need to buy expensive out-of-season fresh vegetables when the price of a head of cauliflower starts to rival that of your child's college tuition. Special supplementation is not required, with the sole exception of vitamin D in the winter, and that's not specific to keto. We should all be taking vitamin D supplements when sunlight is in short supply.

One of the things that dietitians excel at is the counselling and education part of dietary change. As nutrition experts, we are aware of all the elements that inform people's daily food choices: physical, emotional, psychological, hormonal, socioeconomic, societal—bet you didn't realize that so many factors go into what we eat and what we think about what we eat...

The important thing is to begin where you currently are in respect to all of these factors. It's not practical to recommend farm-hopping around the countryside buying premium organic, pastured, blah-blah-blah stuff to someone living on a fixed income, with a family of five and an unreliable car, and who works 40 hours a week to make ends meet. Keto can be done using regular grocery store products, with no expensive supplements, and can be fitted into a household's normal pattern. And fasting is practically free! Yes, it's really different from the Standard American Diet (aptly called the SAD diet) but no, it's not impossible.

Don't let the idea of Perfection get in the way of Progress.

The First Two Weeks –
Building Your Keto Muscle

You will be planning your meals to be based on animal protein foods and vegetables, with enough added fats to satisfy your hunger. This will automatically reduce your carbohydrate intake greatly, not to ketogenic diet levels, but low enough that you will send a metabolic message to your cells. This message will be, "The sugar supply is limited, the fat supply is plentiful, so upregulate your fat-burning metabolic pathways." Whether you actually write out a meal plan or not is up to you—it's a useful tool for some, and others will simply fill their kitchen with allowed foods and see where the spirit leads them each mealtime. Intuitive vs. planned—which kind of food preparer are you?

Making the switch to low-carb eating can be a bit uncomfortable if you've been eating a Standard American Diet and your body is suddenly not getting its usual dose of carbs at the usual frequency. This has been termed "low-carb flu" or "keto flu," as it can feel like flu symptoms. It's partly due to potential electrolyte imbalance (a change in the supply of tiny, electrical-charge-carrying particles) in your blood and tissues. The kidneys will allow a sudden release of fluid bloat with the diet change and electrolytes are lost with this process (as are the gratifying first few pounds of any diet—water weight). Along with the water goes sodium, potassium, and chloride, the main charge-carrying electrolytes. Adding a good salt to your foods remedies this situation for most people. Pink salt, black salt, Celtic sea salt.

"Keto flu" is also a result of your body having only sugar-burning machinery in place inside the cell. Remember that you have the blueprints coded into your DNA for a very efficient fat-burning metabolic pathway but if you have never called on the body to need it, it won't exist yet. The body actively "declutters" any tissues or materials that it has no immediate need for. That's why muscles get smaller and weaker when we don't use them. Once we begin to give our body the signal that we need them (such as when we exercise), the body responds by increasing muscle mass and strength. In the same way, as we give our bodies the signal that we are consuming more fats (by eating more fats and reducing carbs), the body will respond by opening up the DNA blueprints and starting production of the fat-burning metabolic pathways. Once this is in place, keto flu is gone and you achieve Metabolic Flexibility. This is nothing weird—we are all born in ketosis, with metabolic flexibility in place (breast milk is both a high-fat and carb-containing food, after all) and it is our birthright. It's our lifestyle and current diet that has taken it away from most of us.

Foods List:

All unprocessed meats: Beef, all poultry, lamb, pork, goat, rabbit, fish (both freshwater and saltwater—but try to avoid Asian-sourced fish), shellfish, and seafood of all kinds (unprocessed and unbreaded), organ meats. Venison or other game meats. Fresh-made sausage.

Moderate use of processed meats: One serving max per day of bacon, ham, cold cuts, pepperoni sticks, jerky, smoked meats.

Eggs: Chicken eggs, duck eggs. Always include the yolks.

Dairy: Hard cheeses, cream cheese, heavy cream (32%), coffee cream (18%), Parmesan cheese, full fat sour cream (14%), and butter, of course!

Vegetables: All vegetables that grow above ground, with the exception of corn (which isn't really a vegetable anyways...). Moderate use (½ to 1 cup once daily) of below-ground vegetables (carrots, potatoes, sweet potatoes, parsnips, beets, turnip, rutabaga). Onions, including sweet onions, can be used for flavouring and as a condiment.

Legumes: A very small quantity of legumes (dried peas, beans, lentils) can be used in the keto diet, but these podded seeds are high in starch and protein both. Use only occasionally and only a few tablespoons at a time.

Fats: Butter, olive oil, avocado oil, coconut oil, pork lard, bacon fat, beef tallow, ghee. Also, avocado, olives, full-fat mayonnaise, but ideally

THE FIRST TWO WEEKS — BUILDING YOUR KETO MUSCLE

make your own from light olive oil or avocado oil.

Condiments: Mayo, as mentioned above, mustard (not sweet mustards), unsweetened ketchup (in moderation), dill pickles (not sweet pickles), capers. Soy sauce or wheat-free tamari in moderation. Horseradish, wasabi. Balsamic and other vinegars.

Fruits: One serving (½–1 cup) max per day of the following: berries (fresh/frozen, strawberries, blueberries, raspberries, blackberries); fresh cherries (½ cup); small oranges or apples, clementines.

Nuts: Moderate use (1 oz or 30 g) of macadamia nuts, almonds, pecans, walnuts, pistachios. Avoid cashews and peanuts. Raw and unsalted preferred, soaked if desired. An ounce (30 g) or less at a time, as they are very calorie-dense.

Sweeteners: Avoid "keto baking." Use very small amounts of Stevia, erythritol, and monk fruit, and try to use these products only where absolutely necessary, for example, as you transition to unsweetened coffee or tea. Unlearning a preference for sweet tastes is a big part of making a keto diet successful. Totally avoid Aspartame, Splenda, sucralose—anything from a factory, not a plant. And remember that most "sugar alcohols"—the ones ending in "itol"—have nasty gastrointestinal (GI) symptoms if used in quantity. Erythritol is the only one that's relatively mild on the GI tract. For the first two weeks, no "keto" bread or grain alternatives.

Eat enough that you're not hungry. That means eat until full and until you can comfortably go for at least three hours without needing more food. Be sure to add salt to your meals, as you will not be using processed food items that are already salted. Keeping your sodium intake up is important to reduce the discomfort that can come with sudden carbohydrate restriction.

Moving Into Nutritional Ketosis

Getting into nutritional ketosis involves a more restrictive diet than what is listed above. You really can't go straight from the SAD diet into ketosis without being really uncomfortable, so the adjustment period, as outlined above, is the most sustainable way to go.

Ketosis occurs when carbohydrate intake is low enough that the body is forced to make ketones from fatty acids and then use them as fuel in the cells. Blood sugar levels will drop to a low but very stable level, supplying the tissues that prefer glucose as their fuel and insulin levels will be low as there's no large amount of carbohydrate entering the bloodstream at one time. A ketosis-generating level of carb intake is generally recognized as being 20–50 g/day. Although there is some debate about this, the carbs are generally measured as "net carbs," meaning that non-insulin-stimulating carbs, such as those found in undigestible dietary fibre, are not counted. To get this number, calculate as follows:

Total carbs(g) - Fibre(g) = Net carbs(g)

The absolute easiest way to track your net carbs is to use an online or smartphone app such as Carb Manager or Keto Manager. The database in this app is huge and all the math is done for you. It's user-friendly and allows for you to add your own recipes and foods into the database as well. There's a limited free version, a purchased version for a couple of dollars, and a "Premium" version with a monthly subscription fee. The single-time purchase version has everything you will need.

Many types of eating can be ketosis-promoting but not all are healthy and nutrient dense as well. You can get into ketosis by eating nothing but eggs and cheese but that gets boring really fast and is deficient in a variety of nutrients, most notably iron. You can get into ketosis on a vegan diet but it's extremely limiting and highly nutrient deficient. You can eat nothing and end up in ketosis rather quickly. Fasting is powerful but not sustainable as a dietary approach, obviously. That way is called starvation and leads to death…

So a healthy keto diet is one that is nutritionally complete and leads the body into a state of nutritional ketosis, producing ketones and using them as fuel. It also allows for a low circulating insulin level, allowing the use of stored body fat for energy in the form of fatty acids.

Foods List:

All unprocessed meats: Beef, all poultry, lamb, pork, goat, rabbit, fish (both freshwater and saltwater—but try to avoid Asian-sourced fish), shellfish, and seafood of all kinds (unprocessed and unbreaded), organ meats. Venison or other game meats. Fresh-made sausage.

Moderate use of processed meats: One serving max per day of bacon, ham, cold cuts, pepperoni sticks, jerky, smoked meats.

Eggs: Chicken eggs, duck eggs. Always include the yolks.

Dairy: Hard cheeses, cream cheese, heavy cream (32%), coffee cream (18%), Parmesan cheese, full-fat sour cream (14%). And butter!

Vegetables: All vegetables that grow above ground, with the exception of corn. Onions, including sweet onions, can be used in moderation for flavouring and as a condiment. **Avoid starchier vegetables that grow below ground** (carrots, potatoes, sweet potatoes, parsnips, beets, turnip, rutabaga.) **Avoid tubers. Avoid legumes.**

Fats: Butter, olive oil, avocado oil, coconut oil, pork lard, bacon fat, beef tallow, ghee. Also, avocado and olives. Full-fat mayonnaise, but ideally make your own from light olive oil or avocado oil.

Condiments: Mayo, as mentioned above, mustard (not sweet mustards), dill pickles (not sweet pickles), capers. Soy sauce or wheat-free tamari in moderation. Horseradish, wasabi. Balsamic and other vinegars.

Fruits: One serving (½ cup) max per day of the following: berries (fresh/frozen, strawberries, blueberries, raspberries, blackberries). No stone fruit or citrus, other than lemon wedges or juice.

Nuts: Moderate use (1 oz or 30 g) of macadamia nuts, almonds, pecans, walnuts, pistachios. Avoid cashews and peanuts. Raw and unsalted preferred, soaked if desired.

Try to avoid "keto baking," especially anything that uses large quantities of non-nutritive sweeteners as these really don't help with retraining your body to enjoy the taste of fat-rich and satiating foods. There are plenty of recipes for keto alternatives to breads, muffins, cereal, and porridge to be found online and some in the Recipe section of this book. But other than a jam alternative, you won't find recipes here for cookies or cakes. Research is now showing that the body responds to both real sugar and non-nutritive sweeteners with an insulin response, just what we are trying to avoid. Keep this kind of treat for birthdays or Christmas, not every day. The same sweetener rules apply as in the first two weeks.

Create Your Plate

On a nutritionally complete, healthy keto diet, all meals should include an animal-based protein source, a healthy fat source, and enough vegetables to feel satisfied, both physically and mentally/emotionally. In our culture, eating is way more than just fueling the machine, although that's really all it should be. So food needs to fulfill social, psychological, and emotional needs as well. Learning to detach yourself from these other requirements is the topic of other books, but realize that food addiction is real, societal pressures are real, family and emotional food triggers are real. If this statement rings true for you, consider getting some help from a counsellor or clergy to address non-food issues that might be making it challenging for you to eat for your best health. Fortunately, eating a ketogenic diet that minimizes blood sugar spikes is very helpful for reducing the physical cravings of carb addiction, making it easier to stick with the plan.

BREAKFAST:

An optional meal. Wait until your body tells you that it's hungry before eating your first meal of the day. The longer you can stretch the fasted period (since your last caloric intake the evening before) the better. At the barest minimum, make sure that there's 12 hours between evening eating and the breaking of your overnight fast the next morning. So if you finished dinner by 7:00 p.m. on the previous evening, don't start eating breakfast before 7:00 a.m. the next day at the earliest. If you just have a black coffee or tea when you get up, you might find that you don't actually get hungry until 10:00 a.m. or so. Congratulations, you have just completed a 15-hour fast!

Culturally, we have decided that some foods are "breakfast foods" and some are not. In North America, we typically think that bland, sweet grain-based foods are normal—cereal, toast, porridge, biscuits. None of these foods fit into a lower-carb approach. Instead, think about the savoury breakfast options—eggs, sausage, cured meats, such as bacon or ham, cheeses. These are all rich in protein and healthy animal fats and are full of salt and umami-flavour, providing a highly satiating meal.

Of course, any food that fits into a keto diet is acceptable for a breakfast meal. Leftover vegetables and meat? Go for it. To make it a bit more traditional, take those leftover vegetables and meat, chop them up, and use them as the centre of an omelet. Leftover casserole? Perfect on its own. Greek salad? Why not?

If you want a more traditional breakfast, there are "keto baking" alternatives for breads, muffins, cereal, and porridge. They definitely require a bit more planning and food prep but most can be made in quantity to have around for busy days. Several recipes are included in the Recipe section of this book, but the internet is full of keto baking ideas. For best satiety, however, try to stay away from very sweet breakfasts, such as "keto" versions of donuts, Danishes, cinnamon buns, maple syrup, sweet smoothies, or coffee cake.

BREAKFAST IDEAS:

Hardboiled eggs – plain and salted or dipped in mayo or made into devilled eggs.

Fried eggs – cooked in butter, bacon fat, or leftover meat dripping (cooking eggs in the saved fat from frying hamburger patties is delish!).

Poached eggs – sous vide is apparently the bomb for creating perfect poached eggs that you literally cook in their own shell then crack open. But a frying pan of water works fine.

Scrambled eggs – scramble the eggs with added coffee cream, heavy cream, or sour cream, then add salt, pepper, and dill if desired. Cook in an animal fat. Add a bit of cheese while cooking if desired. Three eggs make a hefty mound of eggy goodness.

Omelet – make up and season the egg mix the same as for scrambled, but don't mix it up while cooking. Add filling ingredients on one side of the eggs and allow to cook gently, then fold the eggs over to create a half-moon layered omelet. Allow to cook a bit longer to finish any cheese melting that needs to happen inside the mound. Slide onto a plate and enjoy. Filling ideas: Cheese of any kind, sautéed onions, sautéed or leftover vegetables, spinach, black or green olives, any leftover or breakfast-style meat (bacon, chicken, ham, cooked ground beef). Be creative and open to experimentation. There's not much that doesn't taste good sandwiched inside eggs.

Keto bread or toast – any type of keto bread or buns, warmed or toasted, buttered, topped with cheese, peanut butter (no-sugar type), nut butters, cream cheese, or a savoury type dip or spread. Keto breads can be made as individual servings—keto mug bread recipes abound on the internet—or made ahead in larger quantities (see my Focaccia Bread recipe) and frozen for easy use or purchased (horribly expensive and hard to find).

Breakfast sandwich – of course, keto bread or buns can be used like regular bread to surround a breakfast sandwich, à la Egg McMuffin or Tim Hortons breakfast sandwich.

Keto granola – this is a cold cereal alternative that is based entirely on nuts and seeds. It uses a non-nutritive sweetener and egg whites to provide the sweet glaze and crunch that characterizes regular granola. It's awesomely good but can be hard to limit. I called it Keto Crack-ola for a reason...

Nuts – a modest serving of nuts can make a decent light breakfast, 1–2 oz (30–60 g) of macadamia nuts, almonds, pecans, or walnuts is a great at-work or in-the-car breakfast snack. Clean, discreet, easy to carry, quiet to chew. Get a very small container (such as a mini-plastic container designed for carrying salad dressings or condiments), measure out how many nuts comprise your serving, then use the same container every time you carry nuts. You only have to measure once and you have built-in portion control. My little metal box holds 1 oz of macadamia nuts, a perfect small meal for me, of about 200 calories.

Smoothies – personally, I'm not a fan of smoothies but they are a popular breakfast option, especially for those who must make and run in the mornings. As a liquid meal, they have less satiety impact than solid foods. In addition, they tend to be consumed over an extended period of time so they don't really meet the goal of feasting and fasting. Lastly, they are usually at least somewhat sweet, possibly stimulating an insulin response from your body. It can be challenging to make a keto-compliant smoothie without resorting to highly processed and very expensive protein powders or other non-whole-foods ingredients.

However, for those who like smoothies, the following rules should apply:

1. No bananas! Bananas add the creamy factor and a lot of sugar. Instead, add an avocado. Scoop a full avocado into your blender or use ½ –¾ cup of frozen avocado pieces.

2. Use a small amount of keto-compliant berries—¼ cup should be enough—fresh or frozen.

3. Fresh or frozen spinach is a great addition. If possible, find spinach frozen into small pucks. Each puck is the perfect size for adding to a smoothie.

4. Real cocoa, if chocolate is your thing. Real vanilla, if not.

5. Nut butters. A tablespoon of almond butter adds protein and a rich flavour.

6. As little sweetener as you can manage. Use only keto-approved, naturally sourced sweeteners, such as Stevia, erythritol, monk fruit, or a blend of these.

7. Raw egg – this is controversial, as there's a small but real risk of salmonella poisoning with the use of raw eggs. However, if you know and trust where your eggs come from, wash the shells before cracking and consume the smoothie within an hour or two after it's made, the risk is minimal. Salmonella bacteria can multiply in food that is left at an incubation-promoting temperature for extended periods (over two hours) and it can multiply on improperly cleaned food prep surfaces. This means that any equipment used to blend a raw-egg-containing smoothie must be well washed after use. **If your immune system is compromised (you have a low white blood cell or neutrophil count), use whey protein powder in place of a raw egg.**

8. Full-fat yogurt, unsweetened kefir, Greek yogurt, full-fat sour cream, coffee cream, or heavy cream. Adds protein and calcium in varying amounts depending on what you use. And creaminess, of course.

9. Water or ice cubes to thin down the smoothie a bit. All of the above ingredients are rich and heavy—a little added water both increases the volume of the smoothie and makes it more drinkable. It's not necessarily a virtue to be able to stand a straw in it.

10. Many people use unsweetened almond milk in smoothies. This is okay, as the almond milk is low in carbohydrates but it's also a highly processed product with minimal nutritional value. There is better nutritional value in a real, full-fat dairy product, such as the Greek yogurt, kefir, or heavy cream mentioned above, plus water or ice cubes to thin it out.

11. Supplements. Smoothies can be a good place to hide less-than-palatable supplements such as vitamin D drops, collagen powders, MCT oil or powder. I don't consider any of these necessary, except the vitamin D in some form (pills, chewable tabs (sweet alert!) or drops) during the cold dark months.

Of course, any keto-compliant food can be breakfast. Just try to include an animal-based protein, a source of healthy fats, and enough flavour to satisfy. And eat enough that you can get through four to five hours until your next meal without snacking. With this kind of meal, the mid-morning "hangry" spell will be a thing of the past. Blood sugar levels will be rock steady and your energy level will be stable all morning. You'll be an energized, fat-burning machine!

LUNCH IDEAS:

If you are practicing intermittent fasting and stretching your fast to 16–18 hours, lunch may be your first meal of the day and all of the breakfast suggestions above are valid. However, for many people, lunch happens in the middle of a workday. The timing of the meal is preordained and the amount of time allowed is also limited. Often the meal has to be carried from home or purchased away from home.

Salads. The proverbial "big-ass salad" is a term coined by Mark Sisson, the founder of the Primal Blueprint, and the website, Mark's Daily Apple. The "big-ass" part refers to a meal-sized salad that includes all the protein, healthy fats, and vegetables that one needs for a satisfying and flavourful meal. Build as follows:

1. Greens: lettuce, romaine, kale, spinach, arugula, spring mix—whatever you have.

2. Chunky vegetables: cucumber, carrot, broccoli, cauliflower, peppers, mushrooms, shredded cabbage or Brussel sprouts, bok choy, asparagus—the options are endless but include some for crunchy chewing satisfaction.

3. Animal-based protein source: Leftover or precooked meat, such as thin sliced beef, shredded chicken, canned tuna or salmon, cheese, hardboiled eggs, or any combination of the above. Include enough that the meal is satisfying and fills you up for four to five hours. If you are getting real stomach hunger mid-afternoon, you didn't make your lunch big enough.

4. Healthy fat sources: One of the easiest is to add an avocado to your salad. Because avocado browns very quickly, add it just before you eat lunch. Carrying a paring knife and teaspoon in your lunch pack makes cutting and scooping the avocado easy and clean. A tablespoon of olive oil added to bare greens will coat them and keep them fresh for several days. In this way, you can clean and prep the base of your salad and have it ready to just grab a few handfuls and make your travel lunch quickly. Don't add the salty or vinegary dressing until ready to eat, as these ingredients will wilt your greens and ruin the lovely crunch of your salad. Any salad dressing of your choice that avoids soy oil, corn oil, or canola oil is fine, providing that it isn't sweet. Homemade dressings are best, using good olive or avocado oil and tasty vinegars, but there are good store-bought alternatives as well. Primal Kitchen makes a large variety of salad dressings that use avocado oil as their base.

5. If you are following a more moderate low-carb diet, you can consider adding up to ¼ cup of legumes to your salad for additional texture and protein. Examples are kidney beans, black beans, garbanzos, or lupini beans. These legumes have too many carbohydrates to be used in a stricter ketogenic diet.

Sandwiches. Use anything that qualifies as a sandwich filling—egg salad, tuna or salmon salad, cold cuts, and sliced cheese are all good. Serve in romaine lettuce boats, low-carb wraps, or on low-carb bread. Garnish with sliced onion, non-sweet pickles, mayo, sprouts, or tomato slices.

Soup. A broth-based or creamy soup made with allowed ingredients. Ensure that the soup has some protein and fat content if it's going to be the main course at lunch. Some easy examples would be chicken and vegetable, creamy broccoli with cheese, cream of mushroom, noodle soups made using shirataki noodles. (Shirataki are thin, translucent, gelatinous traditional Japanese noodles made from the konjac yam (devil's tongue yam or elephant yam). They have little to no usable carbohydrate content.)

Casseroles. Great make-ahead options. Prep cook on the weekend and portion into weekday lunches. Again, adequate protein and fat content for satiety lasting four to five hours is a must. Check out the Recipe section for Baked Cauliflower and Cheese casserole or Instant Pot Spaghetti Squash Casserole for great batch cooking ideas.

Takeout. This is a huge subject with enough variations to fill a book. Most fast food options are not made with the best quality ingredients, but it's still possible to stay keto compliant when faced with a strip of fast food restaurants. Probably the best option is a salad with protein.

Subway will make any sub variety into a salad. My favourite is tuna salad with extra bacon. For dressing, I choose mayonnaise and a tiny shot of the sweet onion teriyaki dressing. That allows for mostly full fat dressing, with a wee bit of tang. Like the subs, you can choose whatever toppings you like from their veggie bar and shredded cheese as well. Chicken Caesar salad is always a good choice at restaurants, as long as you specify no croutons. Get bacon crumbles (real bacon only, not the fake stuff) added if available.

Bunless burgers are another popular and widely available choice. Many restaurants will serve their burger in a bowl with shredded lettuce or available toppings. Sides of fries can often be swapped out for a salad at minimal additional expense.

At a Chinese takeout or restaurant, order a main dish of beef and broccoli or basic Chinese mixed veg with almonds and chicken. The sauces have some starch added but generally are not sweet. Avoid anything with noodles, rice, breading, or sweet sauces.

At a Japanese restaurant, miso soup is a good starter, then choose sashimi for the entrée (decline the bowl of steamed rice that comes with most sashimi dinners). This meal is pathetically devoid of any healthy fats (though great for protein) so don't expect to be satiated for hours afterwards.

Smokehouse/BBQ restaurants have wonderful meat-centric meals, but most smoked meat has been either rubbed or marinated in sugar-laden seasoning prior to smoking. And, of course, it's served with very sweet BBQ sauce. The amount of sugar that remains in the smoked meat is generally pretty insignificant compared to the amount of protein and fat that you will be consuming, especially if you choose beef brisket or back ribs. Pulled pork is usually higher in sugar content.

Shawarma meat is pre-seasoned but not sweet. Most shawarma restaurants slice the meat and build your meal after you order, so it's easy to get the meat served without the pita, on or beside a bed of lettuce, and dressed with tahini, garlic sauce (toum), and the assorted vegetables that are usual shawarma condiments. Worst case scenario —unwrap the pita and eat the contents with a fork. Discard the pita.

SUPPER:

Doing a keto diet well generally involves cooking at home. It means starting with basic fresh (as in unprocessed) ingredients and creating the kind of suppers that your parents or grandparents would have recognized, only without the potatoes and bread.

Base supper on meat, lower-carb vegetables, added fats, and low-sugar condiments. There are low-carb recipe alternatives for many traditional suppers available on the internet by simply googling "keto" whatever. Keto breaded fish or keto fried chicken or keto lasagna. Vegetables can be raw, steamed, boiled, oven roasted, barbequed, mashed—whatever your fancy. Adding fats to the vegetables is an easy way to ensure that your meal is satisfying. Butter, olive oil, bacon fat, or full fat sour cream are all options. Be sure that your meal is adequately salted for flavour and mineral content. You can liberally use herbs and spices, hot pepper flakes or hot sauces, mustard (non-sweet varieties such as Dijon), and horseradish to add flavour and interest to your meals.

A quick and easy sauce that we enjoy on pan-fried fish is to mix three parts mayo with one part Dijon mustard, then stir in a teaspoon or two of capers and their pickling liquid. Mixes up in seconds and really elevates a simple worknight supper into something special.

Another useful hack is to mix up a chicken breading using almond flour and a variety of spices. See my KFC copycat recipe in the Recipes section. You can mix it up as needed or make a triple batch and keep it in the freezer in a large Ziploc bag. When you want oven-fried chicken, simply scoop out some of the breading into another Ziploc bag, drop the pieces into the seasoning mix, spread out on an oiled baking sheet or in a large casserole dish and bake the chicken until well done and crispy golden. This works great for chicken thighs or drumsticks or breasts with the skin and bone intact. Seal the original bag up and throw it back into the freezer. It won't have been in contact with raw poultry and will keep for next time.

It should go without saying that dessert is not a necessary part of supper. Dessert is a treat that should be kept for special occasions only—there's no requirement to end a meal with something sweet. Get out of the habit.

When dessert is going to be a part of supper, such as when you have company over, it can often suffice to break up a bar of good quality dark chocolate into small pieces, place it on a pretty plate with some nuts, such as whole pecan halves, and some fresh fruit (perhaps whole strawberries or tangerines), and let your guests pick at it. Serving espresso in fancy tiny cups with warmed cream can also feel like dessert without being a heavy extra course. You could also serve fat bombs, little barely sweet bites of fudgy goodness. A variety of fat bomb recipes are included in the Recipes section.

For a really special occasion, such as a birthday or Christmas, there are lots of recipes out there for "keto baking"—cakes or desserts that are sweetened with non-nutritive sweeteners such as Stevia, erythritol, or monk fruit. There are also easy keto ice cream alternatives, such as Mason Jar Ice Cream listed in the Recipes section. If you're attending an occasion where you'll be the only person present following a keto diet, you might want to find a bakery that does keto baking and buy yourself a single portion of something decadent and sweet. Or pour yourself a coffee or tea, move far away from the buffet table, and find some interesting people to talk to. No matter how you choose to deal with situations like this, go into them with your eyes wide open and a strategy in place. And no matter what, don't arrive hungry! Eat your excellent, satiating keto meal before you go so that there's no chance of being sabotaged by real body hunger.

The Truth About Snacking

How many times a day you eat is entirely up to you but realize that snacking is always an emotional event and that when you are experiencing true hunger, you should eat a satisfying meal. True hunger is triggered by hormonal and blood sugar changes that are a consequence of not eating for several hours. True hunger is not an emotional event. That's the goal, not necessarily where you start. In the beginning, have lots of great keto-compliant snacks around to help you through the tough times. This will include meat-based snacks, savoury/salty snacks, crunchy snacks, and sweet items for desserts.

I used to be a big fan of snacking on fat bombs and pork rinds, cheese "crackers," and "keto baking." Over time, however, I have really let all those things go, as I need much less in the way of snack items to get me through the day. Practicing time-restricted eating helps with that for sure. Having a low-carb cookie or cheesecake recipe in your back pocket is great when you get invited to someone's house for supper, or to a potluck, but shouldn't be part of your everyday eating in the long term.

Start by taking a deeply honest look at what kind of snacking really satisfies you and what part of you is really being satisfied. Are you a stress eater? A boredom eater? Are you having "mouth hunger," "heart hunger," or true stomach hunger? Are you an opportunistic snacker—vulnerable to every environmental cue or trigger that crosses your path?

What kind of snack feeds your soul as well as your body? Do you have a sweet tooth, a salty tooth, or possibly a creamy tooth? Do foods with umami (the earthy richness of cheeses or meats or mushrooms) satisfy you?

Understanding the WHY of your snacking habit or food addiction is the first step in addressing it. Tackling these issues can be hard, as they require honest introspection without self-guilt or blame, just acknowledgement of your needs and coping strategies.

For me, it was always cheese and crackers. Preferably orange cheddar, the cheese of my childhood. I often say that I have never met a cheese that I didn't like but when push comes to shove, it's orange cheddar all the way. With crackers. That combination of rich fattiness, pungent flavour, and salty crunch has been a comfort food for me for decades. Childhood desserts and snacks, university dorm food, afterwork pick-me-up, and after the kids were (finally!) in bed at night. That and a cup of milky tea—heavenly! Once I could identify that cheese and crackers carried with them much more than simple nutritional value, I could make better decisions about when and how much to eat. I was also able to strategize a way to have the same crunch combination in a keto-compliant way. My awesome cracker recipe is included in the Recipe section of this book.

Once you have an awareness of the WHY of your snacking, you can recognize what it is that you're really feeling (boredom, anxiety, stress, neglect, lack of self-esteem), and that's the first step in addressing your real needs in a non-food way. Remember that all learned addictive/out-of-control behaviours are coping strategies that have benefited you in some way in the past. They might no longer be serving your needs or helping you to achieve your goals but they were once very important to you. As such, they can be acknowledged and thanked but then released without you acting on them.

Ideally, the best eating pattern is one of feasting and fasting, meaning that you eat a big enough meal of the right foods to provide satiety for hours, then fast until you are really ready (experiencing genuine stomach/body hunger) for the next meal. Then repeat. Undereating calories at every meal is a sure-fire recipe for disaster—you are not satiated and hence end up looking for snacks in an hour or two. Eating a meal based on protein, healthy fats, and adequate micronutrients provides your body with true satiety, a full feeling in your belly without bloating or pain, and a peaceful lack of interest in continuing to eat. That feeling can last for hours—it's liberating! And quite a revelation for those who have never experienced freedom from food thoughts and cravings.

The Chemo Experience

A few days after New Year's Day 2019, I started chemotherapy. To say that I was scared would be an exaggeration but I was anxious. The very thought of putting poisonous chemicals into my very drug-naïve body made me cringe. The thought of deliberately making myself so sick with side effects was disturbing. The thought of giving up my usually stellar health and strength and becoming frail and vulnerable upset me. It felt necessary but so very wrong on so many levels.

As a health professional, I was not overwhelmed by the nature and process of the big regional Cancer Centre (London, Ontario, in my case) but it is a very overwhelming place nevertheless. You receive a patient number and are then transferred from department to department throughout the day, always identified by that number. It's dehumanizing but essential to the integrity of the system.

Patient numbers and other ID processes are used to ensure that the proper treatment is given to the proper patient. I get that. But it also serves the purpose of distancing the staff somewhat from their patients. They will look at your wristband before ever making eye contact. In fact, there were some members of the staff that never really did meet my eye.

This protects the staff from being absorbed into the anxieties and emotional needs of their patients and I understand that. Health professionals give of themselves all day, every day, in a situation that could easily suck them dry. Burnout is common among nursing staff and others who counsel or care for patients. However, from the other side of the bed, I really wished for a warmer experience from many of the chemo nurses that I met.

They were all competent and exuded a confidence in what they did that was reassuring but would often decline to engage in the kind of small talk or banter that helps to put one at ease.

My chemotherapy days were long. That was by design, since I was having chemo three hours away from home. Rather than have a clinic appointment with the doctor, then come back for chemo in the next day or two, I would smash everything into one long day. We'd stay in a hotel within walking distance of the clinic and were usually finished with breakfast (only coffee for me), checked out, and walking across to the hospital by 7:15 a.m. It was still dark outside at that time, since it was winter. I'd be all ready to go with my health card out when the registration desk opened. Once registered, I'd head off to the lab for blood work, then after that, return to the ranks of chairs outside the clinic to await my doctor's appointment. That was usually an hour or more, since we had to wait for my blood work to be processed and for Dr. S to arrive, usually at around 9:30 a.m.

One of the advantages of all this sitting around was the opportunity to connect with others going through the same process. I met and had meaningful conversations with several women who were travelling the same journey as me, often much further along, and I found them inspiring. One woman, in particular, was there to meet with the social worker and we struck up a conversation. She was on her third recurrence of ovarian cancer. She was about my age, a lovely, calm, and in control lady. As much as I hope to never have a recurrence, I was reassured by her attitude that she was living her life *with* her cancer, not in spite of it.

The clinic visit started with an assessment by the clinic nurse, then there was some more waiting for the oncologist, Dr. S. His visit was often short—he really just needed to check on my response to the previous chemo session before he could confirm the orders for that day's chemo drugs. And since I generally had little to report, other than my less-than-stellar blood test results, he often seemed almost brusque. It was clear from his manner that we weren't going to spend time discussing what happens after chemo. That discussion would wait for a special conference visit at the end of the chemo process. That was hard for me, as I'm a planner.

Despite having my bone marrow depressed by the chemo, I never had blood tests bad enough to require adjustments in timing or dosage of my drug regimen. I had made it clear at the outset that I was willing to accept whatever was best to eliminate the cancer cells from my body on the first go-around. My attitude was: "Hit me with your best shot!" So Dr. S never lingered for long after he'd written the orders for my drugs. I tried several times to tell him about my experience with the keto diet and fasting but he would brush me off with something like, "Different things work for different people—glad it's working for you." I understand that he was unable to get into a discussion about it during his busy clinic day but still I don't ever remember deep concern expressed by him or the clinic nurse.

After clinic, we would head back into the core of the cancer centre, around to the chemo clinic registration area where I would reregister. We were given yet another number (so that the staff didn't call our names out as they collected us for our treatment). Then there was more sitting in waiting room chairs until my number was called. I would be ushered into the chemo suite anytime between 10:00 and 11:30 a.m.

Because of my peritoneal chemotherapy and because I would be there for about seven hours, I was always given a bed rather than an IV chair. Thank goodness for that! Each of the two wings of the chemo suite held about 16 work stations, mostly chairs but also some beds. We all faced each other so there was plenty to watch as other patients received their treatments. Lots of entertainment for a medical nerd like me, watching ports being accessed, nurses gowning and gloving to handle bags of IV solution marked with big biohazard signs, and assessing my roommates for what they decided to wear on their heads and how well—or unwell—they looked.

Some patients would come walking in confidently, kidding and kibitzing with the staff; others arrived looking like they were being ushered to their own execution. Some were wheeled into the suite in transport wheelchairs, too frail to walk; others used walkers for balance or to address their severe peripheral neuropathy—no longer able to feel or control their feet well. Elderly patients would arrive with their adult children accompanying them. There were no children but occasionally I saw young adults with their concerned parents. The most heartbreaking were the elderly couples, looking totally lost and overwhelmed, mere cogs in the giant machinery of the cancer care industrial complex. One day, an old fellow, possibly a farmer, sat next to me with his wife. She likely had never worked outside the home, cooking farmhouse meals and keeping her family cared for, a competent master of her environment and matriarch of her family. Now she had been thrust into the highly disorienting world of a high-tech medical environment, with its endless computers, beeping IV poles, biohazard protocols, and multidrug regimens. And she was trying to support her husband through his equally overwhelming and confusing path, as he negotiated being ill, possible surgeries, strong drugs, and long hallways leading to expensive parking garages. My heart ached for them…

Each chemo cycle would start the night before. They'd pre-load me with the steroids that would help with reducing inflammatory responses to the strong chemotherapy drugs and with reducing the nausea and vomiting side effects. I had to take a large 20 mg dose 12 hours before chemo and again six hours later. I'd set an alarm to wake me up at 3:00 a.m. so that I could get the second dose in on time—not that I was sleeping well anyways. Between the fasting, the strange hotel bed, and the steroids, I was usually wired up and unable to sleep much.

Once I entered the chemo suite, I was given my "pre-drugs," which involved several medications to reduce autoimmune and inflammatory responses to the chemotherapy. During this time, the nurses also gave me a warm gel pack to lie against my arm to bring the big veins to the surface for easier access. The IV setup was put in place—not always easy, as I have small veins. In addition, as chemo advances, the veins get scarred and hardened so accessing them becomes harder after each cycle. Some nurses were very skilled and quickly hit their mark but others not so much…and each attempt would leave large areas of black bruising that took weeks to fade. I looked pretty beat up by the last cycle, with areas of bruising on both arms in various bilious shades of black, purple, green, and yellow.

Forty-five minutes after the pre-drugs, the first chemo drug, Paclitaxel, would be started. First, the nurses flushed my IV, then administered the drug at a mere trickle, just in case of a negative reaction. Then a wee bit more of a trickle, then a bit more. Finally, after three titrations, the real IV rate was reached and then I'd have about three hours of drug administration. During this time, I would knit, watch videos on my computer, listen to books, or work on my blog. Usually, during this lull, Mike would refill my thermos from the coffee shop, then head off to find lunch and do some big city shopping.

At the end of the chemo drug bag (usually a litre), I'd be disconnected from the IV but they'd leave the access port in my arm, just in case. That was my big chance to go to the bathroom free of the IV pole. Last chance, actually, because once the nurse accessed the chemo port on my chest wall for the second chemo drug, I was stuck in the bed for the rest of the afternoon.

The second drug, Carboplatin, was poured right into my abdominal cavity using the chemo port. Because this chemo's job was basically to eliminate any rogue cancer cells that might have been left behind from the cyst rupture and removal, it made sense to put the drug right where these sneaky little escapee cells might hang out. By bathing the outer surfaces of all my internal organs with this drug, getting into all the nooks and crannies of my abdominal and pelvic cavity, I had the best chance of catching any cells that might cause "seeding" of new tumours.

To make this possible, I'd had a chemo port surgically installed under the skin of the right side of my chest, up against my ribcage. It's a little button-like cylinder that can have a short but large diameter needle poked directly into it. From there, a long silicone tube took half a litre of flushing solution down into my pelvis and squirted it out around my bowels and bladder. This was followed by a litre of the chemo drug itself and then another half litre of flushing solution. So in the space of about an hour and a half my belly would be marinated in two litres of fluid. I felt bloated and stuffed with all that liquid floating around inside me. The bed would have to be lowered almost flat for this whole time so I could no longer knit or work on my computer. Usually, I read or played word games on my phone.

The worst part was the last part. Not because it was difficult or unpleasant but simply because it was the last…I had to lie in the bed and "swish" the contents of my belly around, ensuring that the chemo drug got into every little corner of my convoluted insides. The bed was completely flat for this; I had to lie on my right side for 15 minutes, then flip to my left side for 15 minutes, then repeat both sides for a total of one hour.

What made it the worst part? Simply the fact that by the time it came around, I'd been at the clinic for over 10 hours, most of the chemo suite had emptied out, some of the staff had gone home, and the sky outside the windows had become as dark as night again. I just wanted to get the hell out of there. Lying completely flat in the bed on my side meant that most forms of entertainment weren't easily accessible. I was generally exhausted by then and would actually nap for a while. I'd set my phone alarm for every 15 minutes so that I wouldn't have to stay a single minute longer than necessary. The moment my obligate hour was up, I'd look for the nurse to take out the needle and let us go. Usually, we were the last patients there and the lights would be out in the deserted lobby as we left.

So that was my chemo day: Arriving before the clinic opened at 7:30 a.m. and walking out after it had closed, except for the cleaning staff, at about 6:00 p.m. It sucked. Then, of course, we had our three-hour drive home. All of this happened every three weeks in the middle of a Central Ontario winter. At least half of my six cycles took place during winter storms, making driving difficult. I would recline my seat back to make room for my bloated belly and trust my dear hubby to get us home safe. Which, blessedly, he always did.

That first night after chemo was always rough. Despite being exhausted from the previous night's poor sleep, I would only be able to rest for a few hours, then my crampy belly would intrude and make me flop around in bed like a landed fish. That's when I would get up, put on my loose fleece pajama pants, and head downstairs to spend the rest of the night in my recliner, covered with my very special fleece-lined quilt and a prayer shawl, dozing with my legs curled up tight to protect my belly. Mike would usually find me there in the morning.

Counting Cycles

"Today is Day 4 of chemo cycle four, so I am now two-thirds of the way done." Sort of…the world counts chemo that way—the moment that the drug drip stops, you are done with the next cycle. But in real life, that's just the beginning.

For me, each chemo cycle started about three days before the actual day of drug administration. That's when I headed into the lab to get blood work done to determine my response to the previous cycle and whether I'd recovered enough to have the next set of medications. Since all chemo is toxic and causes extensive damage in the body, the effects tend to be cumulative, with each cycle causing a little more of a drop in blood work, a little more damage to tissues, such as nerves and gut linings, and a little more hair loss (mostly noticeable in brows and lashes as time went on).

So sometime on Monday of my chemo week, I would get two vials of blood taken at our local lab, then wait anxiously for the results to be posted online so that I could check them. I read blood work results all the time as part of my work as a Registered Dietitian so I could certainly interpret my own values. The blood values being checked were mostly related to my bone marrow function, liver function, immune function, and overall protein status. I would obsessively reload the lab results page every 15 minutes or so on Monday evenings, even going so far as to take my phone to bed with me so that I could check in the middle of the night to see if they had appeared yet.

On Tuesday of chemo week, I would have a phone call with my clinic nurse, Tanya, who had reviewed the lab results, to discuss their impact on my chemo plans for the week. Even though I frequently had low lab results, we always decided I would go to London and redo the labs on the morning of chemo, in the hope that they would have recovered enough to go ahead with treatment. Worked every time. I rebounded like a boss!

Tuesday evening was my last supper before going into the fasting phase of preparation. I would make sure to have a flavourful and satisfying meal, because once it was done, that was it until Friday…

Wednesday, the day before chemo, was a full fasting day and I consumed only black coffee, various teas, water, and usually two servings of bone broth. By mid to late afternoon, we were driving the three hours to London to our hotel. I'd watch my travel partners have their supper (often delicious shawarma if Mike was with me), while I would take my thermos into the restaurant and sip tea. It really wasn't as hard as it sounds. Once at the hotel, I could warm up my second serving of bone broth and drink it down as my "supper."

Taking the pre-load of steroids totally buzzed me and made it almost impossible to sleep. It also caused my blood sugar to spike, despite the fact that I was deep into ketosis from the fasting at that point.

During chemo day, I was poked for an IV site in my arm, poked again to access the chemo port site on my left rib, and given a bunch of oral and IV "pre-meds" to keep side effects and reactions at bay. That's the actual "Cycle Four" that people think of as "chemo." When a cancer clinic client is disconnected from their drugs on the last day of administration, he or she goes out to the lobby and rings a bell that sits there just for this purpose, and the entire cancer centre erupts in applause. It's supposed to be a significant event—the end of the ordeal.

Well, I can tell you that putting the drugs into my body was just the beginning. Chemo drugs are active in the body for over two weeks, wreaking havoc on multiple systems as they rip through looking for cancer cells to annihilate.

In the first 24 hours or so after chemo, I had to endure a three-hour drive home, freshly loaded with 2 litres (about 2 quarts) of fluid stuffed into the not-nearly-spacious-enough areas around my abdominal organs. The first night at home was usually spent in my recliner, feeling crampy, unable to sleep, but oh so tired. My energy level was low the following day so I would occasionally get up, putz around my kitchen or go to the bathroom, but then I'd have to return to my chair. This is the time that having a "nest" to retreat to, and a loving partner who is just kind of "there," is so important. I would still be fasting at this point so consumed only coffee, teas, water, and possibly one last serving of bone broth.

My 72-hour fast would end with supper on Friday. I would have something flavourful, but really easy, planned for that meal. I was almost reluctant to start eating again, as it felt like the fasting protected me from the effects of the chemo. Any mild nausea that I had to endure always happened once I started eating again, usually Day 3 or 4.

By Days 6–7, my energy level would begin to rise, and I would start looking around for productive things to do. I returned to work on Day 7 or 8, usually with good energy to put in a full day's work. Despite feeling so good (I'm sure as a result of the fasting and my body's state of ketosis), the chemo drug was still present and in force, working under the surface of my awareness. I found this out the hard way by ignoring severe constipation that happened during week two of my first cycle and by being so surprised to find that my immune system labs were way low, despite how good I felt. I hadn't been giving the chemo drugs enough respect—I'm smarter now.

Still, by the end of week two, I was already within a few days of doing labs for the next cycle to start again. And that's when each cycle actually ended for me. When the day came that I rang the bell at the cancer centre, I knew that I was still two to three weeks away from the "End." Once that last few weeks were over and I didn't have to go back, *then* I would feel done. *Then* the hair growth would start up again. *Then* I could start to think about exercising again. *Then* I could start planning what next fall would look like and our travel plans for 2020. *Then* cancer treatment would finally be behind me.

Part 2
What I Learned

Own Your Decisions

"Nothing happens until you decide. Make a decision and watch your life move forward."
– Oprah Winfrey

"When someone makes a decision, he is really diving into a strong current that will carry him to places he had never dreamed of when he first made the decision."
— Paulo Coelho, *The Alchemist*

"Own your decisions." This was a piece of advice given to me by my oncologist, Dr. S. He is a man who practices the "art" of medicine just as much as the "science" of medicine. He sees his job as giving his patients the information to make informed decisions regarding their treatment and their journey, then encouraging them to take ownership of the path that they have chosen.

Cancer is seen as a very complex disease, with thousands of different manifestations. Some tumours are solid, some are not. Some reside in our skin, others in our bones, organs, membranes, muscles, brain, lymph system, or blood. Within each location, the tumour, or cancerous cell, could be one of several different types. It might respond to hormones, it might not. It might be rapidly growing and aggressive, it might be slow growing and minimally invasive. It might cause rapid displacement of other tissue, leading to severe symptoms, or it might be a silent tumour that grows slowly until finally it impinges on something that results in symptoms. Within every tumour, even in the individual cells, there is a myriad of different genetic mutations that are thought to be a part of the damage of the cell. No wonder we don't have a good single path to cancer treatment.

My cancer, ovarian cancer, is one that's considered to be a "whisper-er," with often mild, nonspecific symptoms that are usually brushed off or attributed to something else. Bit of bloating? Well, don't all women have bloating sometimes? Constipation? Probably just part of getting older and less active—should eat more fibre. Occasional pains in the lower abdomen? Must be something I ate…or too much gardening…

In my case, I had noticed that I was thicker in the waist but attribut-ed it to the fact that I hadn't lost my usual 5–8 lbs over the springtime, getting me down to my weight of the previous summer. So my favourite summer pants were too tight to be comfortable when I was sitting down. Well then, I'd just wear stretch pants or capris or a summer dress. Easy to ignore and blame on other factors. Yet how had I failed to notice a lump in my abdomen that, even at the time of diagnosis, was already as long as my hand? In hindsight, there were a few, very little, niggly things that might have triggered me to an awareness of something being "not quite right." A funny feeling when I rolled over in bed at night, the inability to tolerate my favourite hiking pants with the non-stretchy waistband. I ignored them.

However, once faced with the indisputable fact that there's something "wrong" with or "different" about your body, a decision on a course of action must be made. You can't "unsee" something that you have seen. It's not going to go away if you stick your fingers in your ears and start loudly chanting, "La-la-la-la-la-la-la!" with your eyes squeezed shut.

I had a terrible time deciding to have my hysterectomy and complete the "standard of care" for ovarian cancer. I vacillated for days and weeks, worrying about the size of the incision, the pain, how the removal of a large internal organ would impact my other abdominal and pelvic organs and function; what life would be like going forward. My rational mind knew that thousands of women go through a hysterectomy every year and that life goes on just fine without a uterus. But they weren't me.

In a consult visit with my oncologist, Dr. S refused to guide me in any direct way. When I finally said "Yes" to the surgery, it was like the words were being ripped out of me by force, right from my guts, almost burning my mouth. I know that sounds melodramatic but that's what it felt like. I was so conflicted and unsure. Dr. S could see how hard it had been for me to acknowledge that truth and immediately said, "Now, I want you to own that decision. Don't go back and second guess yourself endlessly. Move forward with confidence that you have made the right decision."

Owning your decision means that you have listened to your own body's wisdom, to the whisper of the Universe or God in your ear, to the ideas and experiences of others, and to your own gut. Vacillating back and forth creates huge amounts of stress and washes your entire system with stress hormones. It leads to anxiety, fear, and questioning that can negatively impact on your sleep, your appetite, and your overall energy level.

Making a decision, owning it, and moving forwards with confidence reduces stress hormones and allows the release of the so-called "happiness hormones"—endorphins, dopamine, and serotonin. A sense of purpose, contentment with your present moment, confidence that good things will result from this decision—these are the rewards of owning your decision.

Once I made the difficult decision to proceed with more aggressive surgery, I *did* move forward with the confidence that I had made the right choice. I believe this is a lesson that I will carry into other areas of my life—writing this book was a decision that I made and owned.

Observations on Hospital Food – From the Patient's Side of the Bed

These observations were originally posted on my Primal RD Facebook page just after returning home from my hospital stay for my hysterectomy and abdominal chemo port placement. I have left them in the present tense.

I have just spent four days in a London hospital as an inpatient and what an eye-opener regarding hospital food. I haven't worked in the hospital system for almost 25 years. Here are my observations…

The restrictions around fasting and refeeding for surgery are amazingly relaxed from decades past. Historically, the instructions for any surgery with a general anesthetic were to fast from everything, including water, during the night prior to surgery. This was called NPO—nil per os. Latin for nothing by mouth. And in the hours after surgery, you would be given a clear fluid tray, comprised of unappetizing chicken or beef broth (from a powder, likely), clear juice, Jell-O, and tea. Instead, I was allowed clear fluids until three hours before my surgery so I could have my beloved black coffee up until 9:00 a.m. And despite being in surgery for several hours, I was given a full meal tray for supper, only two hours after arriving back at my room—pork tenderloin with gravy, potatoes, and mixed veg, two dessert choices (fruit and a crumbly square), plus beverages. I managed about three bites and the tea…

Hospital food is still very firmly entrenched in the low-fat paradigm. There wasn't a healthy natural fat to be found anywhere.

Margarine, low-fat Miracle Whip, and Milkettes were available, not even real cream. The meats were served bare of any interesting sauces or creaminess and the veggies were steamed, no butter or salt/pepper. They weren't mushy soft, which was actually good, but naked steamed broccoli needs help.

Once I was identified as eating "keto," the clinical dietitian came to visit me. She agreed that there was very little keto-friendly food on the menu and gave me a sheet of allowed "write-ins," including cheddar cheese packets and hard-boiled eggs so that improved the situation a bit. Luckily, I had come prepared with keto-friendly snacks and some low-carb protein "shakes."

My first breakfast on post-op Day 1 was a total carb fest. Multigrain cereal, juice, muffin, 2% milk, margarine. There was nothing suitable for me except the awful hospital coffee. Once I could make my own menu choices for the next morning, however, my tray looked dramatically different. Two hard-boiled eggs with salt and pepper, plus a packet of Jif Peanut Butter that I just ate off the plastic knife. Better but not great. My big "walk the hall" exercise was a stroll with a kind young nursing student, walking me off the ward to get a real Starbucks coffee!

Once the floor staff knew that I was a dietitian and eating keto, they all seemed to find time to spend in my room, asked lots of questions and were very interested in some of the science and theories of the low-carb lifestyle. I did a fair bit of teaching from bed. After four days, it was great to get home and back to my own kitchen. I am in awe of the great health care that is available to us as Canadians but the nutrition support system in the hospital could sure use an overhaul.

From a nutritional perspective, how you handle a hospital stay depends on whether the hospital has a selective menu or not. The first day of your stay, you'll likely get served the standard tray, but if allowed, you'll be able to choose your meals for the next day. Advocate for your right to choose your own foods. Request the options for gluten-free or diabetic if necessary and ask for help in getting protein and low-carb vegetable options on your tray. Identify yourself as eating keto and request to see a dietitian. You'll then need to stick up for yourself and your way of eating. There's often a write-in list that you can use to boost the variety of available choices, such as cheese packets, hard-boiled eggs, or mayo packets.

But don't expect the hospital to meet your needs even remotely. If you're in the hospital for something scheduled, plan for your support people to bring food in for you and take a bag of keto-compliant foods and snacks with you. This might include nuts, pepperette sticks, your own butter in a small container, and a low-carb meal replacement drink if you expect to be offered Ensure or a similar product. Then shamelessly take advantage of every scheduled visitor to bring you outside meals (bunless burgers, salad bowls, anything homemade) or good coffee.

If your hospital admission is the result of an emergency, your caregiver and your circle of care can be notified and rally to bring in food for you. But for the first day or two, you might be on your own. Remember that you have the power of fasting in your toolkit and eating little or nothing might be better than eating crap from the hospital tray. If you are questioned by concerned staff, just say, "I'm fine. I just don't like this."

And remember that if you're feeling horrible and a little package of a favourite comfort food crosses your path, it's perfectly okay to eat it. There are no hard and fast rules. I was offered a prepackaged, sweet rice pudding on one of my first trays after surgery. You can bet that I ate it. Rice pudding reminds me of my mom.

Love Your Body – Love the Cancer: It's You, Only Different

As I have travelled this new road called Cancer, I have realized that there are many ways to approach the journey. Nobody asks to take this road—it's full of unknowns, including how long the road will turn out to be—but we are never given the choice. We are simply thrust upon it by the words, "You have cancer." POW! Suddenly, everything you thought you knew about your road ahead has vanished in a puff of smoke, and you've been plunked down in the middle of a deep, dark forest, on a pot-holed, twisty trail with no idea of where it leads.

Sitting down in the middle of the trail for a good cry is a fairly common first choice of action, but it's not going to be a functional plan going forward. Eventually, you have to get up, dust off, and start moving down the trail. But the ground under your feet is no longer as secure as you once thought it was. Puddles, rocks, tripping roots, sudden forks, possible side trails, maybe lots of alluring guideposts—but do you trust them?

Some will travel this road almost paralyzed by fear. They'll spend so much time looking at their feet that they'll have no idea what's around them or up ahead. This is the "victim" mentality. They feel powerless, weak, susceptible to whatever others tell them is the right thing to do. They lose their sense of self in the role of "victim," some willingly, others without realizing it. They might spend time dwelling on why this happened to them, looking for something to blame, whether that's something of their own creation, like a bad habit or toxic emotions, or something outside themselves, like an environmental exposure or something in their medical history. Some people with this mentality stay in that space for their entire journey—it's comforting to not be in charge, to give up control to those they believe are smarter or better equipped to handle their cancer. For others, their mentality evolves over time as they work through the stages of grief or find effective coping mechanisms.

Others will "gird their loins," put a fierce look on their faces, and pick up their "weapons" to do battle with this evil entity that has invaded their lives. They consider the cancer to be an enemy, something foreign and grotesque that has taken up residence in their own precious flesh. This is the "battle" mentality. Everything becomes part of the "fight." Society has decided that we must "do battle with cancer" so this is a socially accepted (even expected) path. The "warrior" persona is one that we see in many YouTube videos and Facebook posts. However, as anyone can tell you, being in a state of constant battle readiness can be exhausting and raises the possibility of all kinds of stress-related negative health consequences.

I have decided on a different path. I look on my cancer as a part of me, only different. Just because something is damaged doesn't make it terrifying or evil. It's just damaged. Most damaged things, whether they be inert objects or emotions or people, are really just in need of being fixed, repaired, healed. In many cases, if we put the right conditions in place, these things will fix or heal themselves. Here's an example: A cut finger doesn't become an intact finger because you put a Band-Aid and some ointment on it. The washing of the wound, the ointment, and the Band-Aid only serve to put the conditions in place for your body to make new tissue and heal the wound. The healing happens from inside—only one tiny bit of the awesome majesty that is life.

Every night since finding out that the cyst that was removed from my body was cancerous, I have gone to bed and placed my hands over my lower abdomen in the heart shape that your thumb and index finger make, consciously giving love to my belly. Yes, there's the possibility that there are rogue cancer cells floating around in my abdominal cavity, but they are ME, a lost and misguided part of me that either needs to be healed back into wholeness or, more likely, must be encouraged to die a cellular death (called apoptosis), also a normal part of what our bodies do to stay healthy. The chemotherapy drugs find these cells (they're drawn to them by their metabolic activity) and encourage them to self-destruct by doing enough damage that the cells recognize they are no longer viable. Then the cellular breakdown and cleanup mechanisms swoop in and mop up the mess, like a team of janitors and maintenance staff. It's an elegant system and another part of the awesome majesty of life.

So I don't consider it a battle. And I'm sure as heck not a victim. I have all kinds of awesomeness inside this wonderful body of mine and I am going to use all of it to help the cancer to disappear. As Marie Kondo (the decluttering guru and author of *The Life-Changing Magic of Tidying Up*) would say, "If it doesn't spark joy in you, thank it for its part in your past life and let it go."

Thank you, CANCER, for your part in my life, bringing me to this point, but now it's time for you to go.

Fat-Adapted/Ketosis/Fasting – The Terminology

Time for a bit of a biology lesson. The terms "fat-adapted," "fat-burning beast," "in ketosis," and "ketogenic" are thrown around a lot in the low-carb community. They can be confusing in terms of what they really mean and what the differences are.

In evolutionary terms, we are designed to carry extra energy around in the very efficient form of body fat stores. Like all mammals, we store extra fat in little pouches called vesicles inside of our cells. We have cells specialized to many different functions and the ones that are designed to store our excess fat energy are called adipocytes. They tend to be found just under our skin and around the organs in our abdominal and pelvic cavities. Fat storage under the skin is called subcutaneous fat and fat storage in our abdomen is called visceral fat. Whether fat cells are accumulating fat or releasing fat is determined by hormones, protein messengers that circulate around in our blood in response to signals from the control centres in our brains. How many fat cells each of us carries is determined by factors in our development. Babies have more fat-cell development in their first year of life, and it's also possible that fat cell creation increases during puberty. Scientists thought that the number of fat cells was a constant in adulthood and they could empty out but never be gone, but with a newer and greater understanding of apoptosis, or programmed cell death, it is now understood that empty adipocytes eventually are broken down and reabsorbed. The body doesn't hang onto what it doesn't need.

We have the ability to burn fat for fuel, either from our dietary intake or from our body stores. We do this by breaking down triglycerides (the storage form of fats—both from our adipocytes and from our diet) into three fatty acid chains and a glycerol backbone. This breakdown takes place in the fluid (called cytoplasm) of each cell in our bodies. The fatty acids are further broken down into small energy molecules called Acetyl-CoA, which is used by the Krebs cycle, the basic energy-producing engine in the mitochondria of cells. The process of breaking down fat molecules for energy production is called lipolysis ("lipo" refers to lipids or fats, and "lysis" means breakdown or destruction). The process is called fatty acid oxidation or beta-oxidation.

We also have the ability to use carbohydrates for energy production, again breaking them down into Acetyl-CoA for use by the mitochondria. This is a simpler and quicker process, providing us with instant energy, a good thing if we need to flee a life-threatening situation. We store a small amount of carbohydrate energy in our liver for use in maintaining blood sugar levels and in our muscles for an instant response to an adrenaline rush (the aforementioned life-threatening situation). But in nature, we were never exposed to the huge amounts of carbohydrates that our current diet provides and our metabolic pathways were never designed to manage such an overload of carbs. Our ancestors would have a large carb feed during berry or fruit harvest season, or when they robbed the occasional beehive, but daily bread or candy were not part of their lives.

When we eat a large load of carbohydrates, extra carbs are transported to the liver and used to create triglycerides for more effective storage. In evolutionary terms, this was an excellent practice. We see it today in hibernating bears who gorge on fruit during the summer and fall, growing huge fat stores that allow them to live through the winter without any additional food intake. We also see how domesticated animals being fed high carbohydrate feeds are unnaturally fatty, from our cattle, to our foie gras geese, to our pets.

When we reduce the excessive carbohydrate content of our diet using a lower-carb approach, we allow the body to use its own fat stores as energy. When carbohydrate intake is consistently low, the cells will recognize the need to create more of the metabolic pathways necessary to break down fatty acids into Acetyl-CoA. This process is called "becoming fat-adapted."

Keto "flu" happens when the body's carbohydrate supply has been drastically reduced but the cells have not yet "upregulated" the production of the fat-processing molecules. What does keto flu feel like? Just what you would expect with an energy supply problem—fatigue, headache, sleeplessness, brain fog, and a sudden precipitous drop in exercise tolerance. It can also be felt in the digestive tract as the body adjusts its digestive processes to deal with increased fat intake. This can reflect in short-duration nausea, constipation, or diarrhea. All of these problems generally resolve themselves in a few days as the body reads the incoming signals (more fat, less glucose coming in) and adjusts the processes accordingly. Think of it as a factory. If the raw materials coming in are oranges, the factory will make orange juice. If the raw materials change to lemons, they will rejig and start making lemonade. It takes an adjustment to the machinery and the basic process. That's how it works in the digestive tract and in each cell. When the body's carbohydrate intake is reduced, new digestive enzymes are produced and new metabolic pathways are created in the cells. Remember that the body does not keep unnecessary junk around so if they aren't needed, cellular components will be broken down and their energy and components reused. That's the process of autophagy (literally: self-eating).

When there is an overabundance of Acetyl-CoA, beyond what the Krebs cycle in the mitochondria can handle, the excess is shunted off to another metabolic pathway that creates ketone bodies. These are molecules that can be circulated in the blood (they are water soluble, unlike fatty acids) and can be used throughout the body as an alternative fuel source in place of glucose. The main ketone body is called beta-hydroxybutyrate (BHB). It can be further metabolized to form two other ketone bodies: Acetone (the fruity smell in the breath) and acetylacetone (excreted through the kidneys and measured using urine Ketostix). BHB is the most abundant ketone and the one that is measured by blood tests.

Ketone bodies can be rapidly processed back into Acetyl-CoA for use in the mitochondria throughout the body. In fact, ketones are the preferred fuel for the brain, as they are estimated to be more efficiently burned than glucose. That's important because our big beautiful brains are energy hogs, consuming up to 20% of our entire energy needs. And when in ketosis, 50%–70% of the brain's energy will come from ketones.

The remainder of the brain's energy needs and the energy needed by red blood cells and the liver must be provided as sugar (glucose) and are supplied by a process called gluconeogenesis ("gluco" means sugar, "neo" means new, and "genesis" means creation). Using protein from the diet, glycerol from the breakdown of fatty acids and lactate from the muscles as building blocks, the liver creates new glucose molecules to meet these needs. Thus, despite having some cells that are obliged to use glucose, we actually have no need for carbohydrates in our diet. We can make everything we need in this elegant system.

When we fast or abstain from any significant caloric intake for an extended period of time, our metabolism shifts towards use of fat stores for fuel. This happens to a mild extent every night when we go without eating for 8–10 hours. As the processing of our last meal is completed, the protein, fat, and carbohydrate absorbed from the digestive tract have been transported to the liver and, according to hormonal signalling from the master glands in our brains, we have either burned them for fuel or used them as building blocks for other needed body materials—both structural (cells, bones, etc.) and functional (enzymes, genetic material, etc.) The excessive carbohydrates (sugar molecules from dietary sugars or starches) that can't be used for fuel immediately will be processed into fatty acids, added to a glycerol backbone, and sent out to the fat stores as a triglyceride molecule. Dietary fats will also be sent out for energy burning in the body cells if there is a low-carb intake but sugar will be burned preferentially. In that case, dietary fats might end up in fat stores as well. Protein, meanwhile, is used for structural material, building, and repair.

During the fasted period, the hormones that have caused all of this storage activity will drop and a different metabolic pattern will emerge. Now the fat cells are not being called upon to accept deposits of fats. Instead, they are being stimulated to release fats into the bloodstream for transport to muscle tissues and other cells where they can be broken down and used as energy. In addition, the fat molecules are called back to the liver for production of ketone bodies to help with fueling the brain and red blood cells. As the fatty acids get broken into ketone bodies and Acetyl-CoA, their glycerol backbones are processed into brand new glucose cells to feed those obligate glucose-burners.

Although this is only a high-level overview of what is happening metabolically in ketosis and fasting, it helps to see the elegance of the system.

Our huge, energy-hungry brains can never be left without enough fuel. If they were, we, as a species, would have just curled up and died every time there was a food shortage. Instead, we have this wonderful, steady supply system that allows us to maintain the vast metabolic machinery that is our brain. Understanding the efficiency of this system will allow you to feel confidence in using a ketogenic diet, the ketosis state and fasting as powerful interventions for good in your cancer treatment.

Cancer Is a Metabolic Disease

In my previous 30 years as a dietitian, I have had little to do with cancer. Instead of considering it a disease that we could impact with nutrition, we saw it as an independent condition that we had to support people through, a strictly reactionary approach. Dietitians would consult with patients who had weight loss or poor food intake related to cancer or cancer treatment effects and teach them a "high-protein, high-energy" diet. In the heyday of the low-fat movement (basically from the 1970s until now), it was almost "naughty" to be telling cancer patients to use extra fat to boost up the calorie content of their food while not impacting on the total volume of food required, since many cancer patients were dealing with small appetites, early satiety, taste changes, nausea, and vomiting. We also pushed a lot of sugar intake, as this would also boost caloric intake without increasing food volume.

After turning my back on the conventional wisdom about moderation, the notion that sugar is harmless and an irrational fear of dietary fat, I wasn't about to buy the party line about cancer any more than I did for type 2 diabetes or obesity. So off I went into the scientific literature.

And lo and behold, I found out that there's a whole body of science that supports looking at cancer not as a genetic disease but as a metabolic one. A disease of disordered metabolism that is similar across many types and locations of cancer. And a disease that has been increasing rapidly in recent years, in lockstep with the increase in other "lifestyle diseases"—obesity, metabolic syndrome, pre-diabetes, type 2 diabetes, coronary heart disease, strokes, ADHD, PCOS, and many other inflammatory processes in our bodies. A study released in the UK in 2018 looked at cancer incidence (how much cancer was diagnosed) between 1980 and 2013 and found that all types of cancer increased in incidence, ranging from uterine (67%) to melanoma (375%) (9). A US review article from 2015 predicted that the number of cancer cases in the US will have increased by about 20% between 1975 and 2020, although much of that will be a result of population aging and growth.

I found out that the original research on cancer metabolism was carried out in the 1930s by a German researcher named Otto Warburg. He was awarded the Nobel Prize for Medicine and Physiology in 1931 for his work discovering and describing the metabolism of cancer cells and what he called "cellular respiration."

Several major world events intervened to cause all of Dr. Warburg's work to be forgotten and mothballed. Not least was the Second World War, which Germany lost. His work was considered so important that the Nazis were willing to overlook the inconvenient fact that he was half Orthodox Jewish but this very association worked against him and his reputation after the war (11).

Moreover, the discovery of DNA, the double helix of life, and the soon-to-follow discovery that cancer had genetic abnormalities, sent the entire machinery of the cancer industry in the direction of genetics and metabolism was forgotten. It is only in the last 10–20 years that researchers have again visited the science around cancer metabolism, looking at these energy and mitochondrial abnormalities as being widespread in many types of cancers, thus providing a new target for treatment. A *New York Times* article in 2016 referred to this science as "An Old Idea, Revived: Starve Cancer to Death" (11).

In normal cells, energy is produced in the organelle called the mitochondria in a series of chemical steps called the Krebs cycle. Scientists around the world today are working on clarifying and explaining the mechanisms of cancer metabolism and how it differs from healthy cells. Electron microscopy shows that the internal structures in the mitochondria of cancer cells are deformed. The process of breaking glucose into energy, a very efficient process in healthy mitochondria, is missing in cancer cells. Instead, the cell uses the ancient process of fermentation, which takes place in the cytoplasm (fluid) of the cell. Fermentation is an inefficient producer of energy. Its by-product is lactic acid. This acid is pumped out of the cancer cell through its membrane, turning the immediate area around it into an acidic microclimate, causing inflammation. Whereas one glucose molecule will produce 36 ATP molecules (adenosine triphosphate, the basic energy currency of the cell) in the Krebs cycle, the by-products of which are carbon dioxide and water, and are clean burning and efficient, fermentation, on the other hand, creates only 2 ATP molecules from a single glucose molecule and its by-product, lactic acid, causes it, basically, to poison itself. Fermentation in the presence of oxygen is a very abnormal process but this is what fuels cancer cells.

Cancer cells generate energy from glucose, not fatty acids or ketone bodies, our other readily available fuels. And because cancer cells have no ability to down-regulate themselves—no "off" switch—they are HUNGRY for glucose all the time. They have more insulin receptors on their cell membrane surfaces than regular cells, ready to pull in any available fuel. They LOVE it when we eat lots of carbohydrates and our blood sugar rises and our insulin levels rise in response.

This is a pretty simplified overview of the basic theory of cancer as a metabolic disease. The feeling among cancer metabolism researchers is that the *genetic* abnormalities of cancer are more likely to be a downstream effect of the disordered *metabolism* than the original cause. There are no definitive answers yet to many of the questions regarding the origins of the genetic damage but it's not important in this discussion. What really matters is that we have the power, through our food choices, to impact on the fuel environment of the body and thus the cancer cells.

Modern North American eating patterns are based heavily on processed products of the industrial agricultural complex. Corn, wheat, soybeans, and canola form the basis of most of the processed foods in our food supply. They lend themselves well to industrial farming practices of monocropping, heavy chemical use of fertilizer and pest control and large machinery seeding and harvesting, making them very profitable to the seed companies and the chemical companies, if not to the farmers themselves. They are processed to create manufactured proteins (soy protein, wheat gluten), manufactured carbohydrates (corn starch, wheat flour, high fructose corn syrup and a myriad of other forms of sugar and modified food starch) and manufactured fats (corn oil, soy oil, canola oil, vegetable oils, margarine, Crisco). None of these foods was part of the traditional human diet before the last 120 years, with the exception of ground whole wheat.

Over the 2.5 million years of human development, the human race, our predecessors, and we ourselves, *Homo sapiens*, have been scavengers, hunters, trappers, gatherers, and fishermen. We ate what we could find in nature. Animals that other animals had killed and left, animals that we were able to bring down ourselves, fish and sea creatures that we could hook or spear or catch with nets, and bugs. Probably lots of bugs, at times. We were the primates who hunted and the primates who tamed fire and learned to cook, making food much more biologically available. Most of the energy contained in plants, in the form of cellulose, was biologically unavailable to us without processing of some kind—soaking, pounding, drying, slaking (with minerals such as lime), and cooking with heat—as our carnivore-like digestive system could not process it. Roots and tubers were modest sources of starchy carbohydrate energy but were only available at a certain time of the year and most of them were tough, fibrous, and bitter with antinutrient phytochemicals. They were starvation-prevention foods but not ever the preferred choice. Fruit was available in abundance for only a short period of the year when the plant produced its seeds, surrounding them with sugar-containing pulp to encourage animal consumption and the spread of their precious seed to other locales through feces drops. Gorging during these brief sugar abundance periods would fatten up the animals that ate them, readying them for the scarcity of winter.

In the last 10,000 years or so, humans have also become farmers and herders, domesticating both animals and some plants to do our bidding. This was an enormous advancement, reducing our dependence on the availability of wild game or the seasonal nature of wild plants. Now our animals were close at hand and could provide us with meat, eggs, and milk on demand. Milk and eggs entered the human food supply for the first time. The first food processing was likely drying meat for storage, salting meat or seafood when salt was available, and processing milk into cultured milk products, such as cheese, kefirs, and yogurt products using bacteria.

As plants were domesticated and gradually hybridized to allow for increased yield, our ancestors learned to store plant foods for consumption during the between-harvest periods. Grains were domesticated from wild grasses, threshed to remove the kernels from the stalks, and then stored in granaries, where they were protected from the environment and from pests. Tubers such as wild potatoes were dried by the ancient peoples of South America and then stored for use during the winter months. Eventually, legumes such as beans were also domesticated, with the dried beans collected from their pods and stored. In order to be fit for human consumption, these agricultural plant starches required extensive processing, such as grinding, soaking, slaking, and cooking to release their nutrients for human use.

In the last 100 years or so, we have become chemists and industrialists. Instead of using basic elements such as water, heat, or salt to change our foods, we have developed the ability to use chemical solvents, deodorizers, desiccants, and artificial flavours and colours to create what writer Michael Pollan termed "food-like substances"(12). This has made it possible to use the products of industrial monocrop agriculture—corn, soybeans, wheat, canola—to create substitutes for our naturally occurring foods. Vegetable oils replacing lard and beef tallow. Margarine replacing butter. Soy protein isolates replacing meat. These bear little resemblance to the food of our ancestors and our bodies really don't know what to do with them. We have also developed hybridization to create plants that produce vastly more sugar or starch than their predecessors. There's nothing about a modern peach or apple or head of corn that resembles their ancestor plants. In *In Defense of Food: An Eater's Manifesto*, Pollan reduces his recommendations to seven words: "Eat food, not too much, mostly plants." In other words, real food, not manufactured food-like substances.

Even more recently, we have developed the ability to modify genetic material, and plants are now being cultivated and sold in the human food supply that have never existed before. The vast majority of the corn (92%) and soy (94%) grown in North America are now genetically modified organisms (GMO). Most GMO technology has been developed to allow the spraying of these crops with herbicides and pesticides without killing them. So on top of it being an unrecognizable genetic organism, it's also bathed in chemicals that have never before been part of our food supply (13, 14).

In the vast scheme of time, the last 10,000 years of domesticated agriculture is a short minute and the age of industrialization is the blink of an eye. Our bodies are still mostly the same as our ancient ancestors'. When we take this magnificent machine that nature has crafted, with its short but efficient digestive tract, huge brain, sharp, forward-focused eyes, and upright posture and feed it chemicalized crap from a factory for decades at a time, it's no wonder that chronic disease, including cancer, develops. When our diets contain little more than highly processed, quickly digested carbohydrates in quantities that our bodies have never experienced before, our hormonal balance gets overtaxed and disease results. When we supply ourselves with chemically modified fats that are not recognizable by the body, our cells do not have the appropriate raw materials to build new cell walls or cellular components. When we mistakenly refuse to give our body natural fats and cholesterol, the basic building blocks of all cell membranes in our body, is it any wonder that cellular malfunction occurs?

I was educated to be a dietitian in the early '80s, when the concept of cholesterol and saturated fats being the ultimate evil was considered the truth and cutting-edge science. I was expected for decades to advise and teach my patients and clients to avoid cholesterol-containing foods, eschew eggs and red meats, trim the fat off all animal products, and avoid full-fat dairy like it was poison. This position still permeates most of the establishments and institutions that give dietary recommendations to the masses, including governments and large disease-based organizations. And yet chronic disease has increased its prevalence exponentially in the past 40 years. There's no denying that heart disease, cancer, Alzheimer's disease, and type 2 diabetes were almost anomalies in the previous centuries to ours. Although we are all living longer than our predecessors, our healthspan is not keeping up with our longer lifespan. We spend decades of our later years unwell. It surely comes down to a question of quantity vs. quality (9).

How could the very foods that had allowed humans to develop as the most successful species on the planet suddenly be so bad? How could meat, fish, birds, animal fats, tubers, nuts, and seeds be so very evil when we have literally achieved planetary mastery by using them as our fuel supply?

The incidence of cancer in the past 100 years has risen dramatically. Yes, more of us live longer now that infectious diseases have been removed as a major cause of death and diagnosis is much more accurate in recent decades. One reviewer in the UK has stated that about two-thirds of the increase in cancer incidence is attributable to longevity but, importantly, the remaining third is caused by lifestyle choices and other factors (9).

What lifestyle factors have changed in 100 years? Lots, obviously. We are hugely less physically active than our great-grandparents. Everything from transportation to housecleaning to our work lives has been changed and made less physically taxing through technology. We live in a world of chemical exposure unlike anything in human history. But we also live in a cleaner world in terms of exposure to indoor cooking smoke and coal-fired heaters. We have a hugely reduced exposure to "filth" of all kinds, living in a hygienic bubble of our own making. This has reduced the epidemics of infectious diseases but also seems to have made us less resilient to environmental stressors—more fragile, in a way (16).

There's no denying that our food supply has changed too. The signals that we put into our body via our digestive tract, the type and proportion of fuel energy we supply, and the chemical/toxic burden of our food have all drastically changed in the last century. Our great-grandparents ate mostly organically grown and raised food, in minimally processed form and often with its natural microbiota intact. The family farm was a closed system, producing its own food—both plants and animals—and also producing the fertilizers required to grow and raise them. Most non-farming households purchased basic staples and raw materials and created their meals from scratch. Think of the roast chicken or roast beef with potatoes and gravy for Sunday dinner. Think of the freshly pulled garden carrot, wiped off on the leg of the dirty work pants of your grandfather and consumed using the same unwashed hands that pulled it out of the ground. Think of eating fresh but unwashed raspberries from a bush at the side of a trail or road. Think of the salamis hanging in the chimney of an Austrian farmhouse, taken down and sliced for a meal. All these foods contain a multitude of naturally occurring bacteria and yeast that have been part of our intake for millennia. Now we can buy a special chemical bath for soaking our produce to remove any trace of other life.

The good news is that with our recent understanding that the cancer cell has a metabolic abnormality and that it is standard across most types and locations of cancer means that we can use metabolic strategies to impact on its growth and strength. Simply by changing how we fuel our bodies, we have nontoxic but very powerful tools at our disposal. Let's look at the significance.

What This Means for Cancer Treatment

Cancer therapy is broadly referred to as "cut, burn, and poison." This refers to surgical approaches, radiation therapy, and chemotherapy. There has been little real change and no major advancements in cancer treatment in decades. The mapping of the human genome, followed by mapping the "cancer genome," has not proven to change the effectiveness of current treatments. Trying to target certain genetic abnormalities with targeted therapies has mostly proven ineffective. Immunotherapy and gene-splicing technology, such as CRISPR, is in its infancy and has not yet been proven effective (17), Research and clinical observation have now shown that all cancers have a wide variety of genetic mutations and mistakes. There's no homogeneity (sameness) between different cancers or even within cells of the same tumour (18). It's like trying to stick a patch over one hole of a colander and expecting to change the rate of water passing through. The entire machinery of the cancer care industry over the past 80 years has been focussed on genetic abnormalities but success has been elusive. No wonder, knowing what we now know about the *heterogeneity* of cancer cell DNA.

But there is some encouraging news: As research into cancer-specific metabolism progresses, it becomes clear that cancer has an Achilles' heel, a weakness that can be exploited. Cancer *needs* sugar. It can't grow and multiply as readily without a steady supply of sugar. Research suggests that up to 80% of cancers have this unusual metabolic pattern. (Some tumours can use the amino acid glutamine as an alternative fermentation fuel, but it's hard to control this in the body, as it's the most common of the amino acids (protein components) and is used in a wide variety of body processes.)

Cancer cells have an increased number of insulin receptors on their surface to encourage insulin to latch on and allow transport of sugar into the cytoplasm of the cell. More insulin circulating in the blood is a good thing for them. More insulin attached to their receptors means that more sugar can enter the cell for use as fuel for uncontrolled growth. Lower insulin levels in the blood means less insulin to attach and transport sugar and therefore less fuel for growth. This stresses the cancer cells and slows the process of cell division and growth.

Metabolism of fatty acids and ketone bodies can only take place in the mitochondria, not the cytoplasm of the cell. Since cancer cells have messed up mitochondria, they can't use these alternate fuels. When insulin levels are low in your blood, they are stressed by lack of access to their preferred fuel but further hampered by the inability to use the prevailing fuel sources (fatty acids and ketone bodies). This is bad for the cancer cells and good for us.

Most of the cells in our body have mitochondria that function just fine, thank you very much, and they are happy to use fatty acids and ketone bodies for fuel. A few cells do not have mitochondria (red blood cells being the prime example) and they require sugar as their only fuel. Luckily, we have a great regulatory system for keeping our blood sugar at a steady baseline level and a backup system for creating glucose, our blood sugar, when we need it. This process is called gluconeogenesis, meaning "creation of new glucose." The substrate, or building material, for making glucose is either amino acids from the muscle tissue or from the diet, glycerol from the breakdown of fatty acids, or lactate from the muscles. Our bodies also store some glucose in our liver in the form of glycogen, a storage starch, for keeping blood sugar levels stable between meals. There's additional glycogen storage in our muscles, ready for fast release into the bloodstream in times of adrenalin response or excessive effort. We carry about 500 calories of stored sugar in our livers and about 1,500 calories in our muscles at any one time.

Two thousand calories max. Compare that to about 3,500 calories of energy stored in every pound of body fat. Even a slim athlete carries around tens of thousands of calories of energy, ready to be used if the conditions are right to allow them to be accessed. What conditions are those? Well, the same conditions that stress cancer cells—low circulating insulin levels.

How's that for a serendipitous coincidence?

It is noteworthy that we are unable to have a blood sugar count of zero—that way lies death! You cannot starve cancer cells by having *no* blood sugar. But low and steady blood sugar, coupled with low levels of the hormone that makes blood glucose available to cells, namely insulin, make it harder for cancer to get enough fuel to happily multiply.

What this means is that we can weaken cancer cells through our food choices. We can also support and strengthen our healthy tissues by the same dietary choices, taking advantage of the metabolic flexibility of normal cells to use fuel sources other than sugar for their energy needs. A weakened, stressed cancer cell is more susceptible to the damaging impact of chemotherapy drugs or radiation energy. A weakened cancer cell can't grow and create the conditions for cell division as effectively as a healthy cell, and it can't stimulate the growth of new blood supply by sending out growth signals that encourage new blood vessel development. Without a supply of oxygen and nutrients being delivered by blood vessels, cancers cannot grow. Slowing this process of angiogenesis (new blood vessel creation) slows the growth of cancer and can even lead to tumour shrinkage. Some chemotherapy drugs, called antiangiogenic drugs, work this way. Wouldn't it be cool if we could have the same effect simply by improving our food choices?

We can! Using a well-formulated, whole-foods-based ketogenic diet creates the conditions for supporting healthy tissue with great fuel and nutrients while stressing glucose-hungry cancer cells. Exaggerating this effect with the use of strategic, therapeutic fasts is even more powerful. That's what the rest of this book is about—putting the power of nutrition into the hands of the person travelling the cancer journey.

The Power of the Targeted Fast for Chemotherapy

There is a growing body of research that looks into the effects of carbohydrate restriction on cancer development and cancer treatments. There is less research focussed on the role of fasting in cancer care but some work has been done by Dr. Valter Longo in California. In 2009, he published a case series report of 10 human patients using fasting during chemotherapy treatments and their response to the treatments. Almost without exception, his patients experienced fewer side effects from the chemotherapy when they fasted than when they ate as much as they wanted.

His work to determine the response of fasting on cancer continues to this day. A more recent article, published in 2018, showed that a fast of 36 hours pre-chemotherapy and 24 hours after had a significant effect on the quality of life for 34 patients undergoing chemotherapy for either breast or ovarian cancers (19). These patients agreed to fast for 60 hours for three of their chemo cycles and eat normally for the other three. After reading about their experiences, when it came to my own treatment, I refused to subject myself to the potential for additional side effects, such as nausea, vomiting, mouth sores, cramping, and muscle and joint aches.

Fasting is like a superpower when it comes to chemotherapy. But to understand this, you need to understand how chemotherapy works. Chemotherapy is simply a drug or combination of drugs, a chemical that's put into your body and that circulates in your bloodstream looking for its target. It's not a precisely targeted "smart bomb," heading only for the tumour cells. Instead, most chemo drugs are aimed at cells that send out the signals of fast metabolism. Remember that one of the hallmarks of cancer is that it has no "off" switch—it's broken—and so it's always in growth mode. Many of these chemicals work by finding and disrupting specific chemical reactions in cellular function that will interfere with this growth.

Some medications will impact on the tumour's ability to convince the body to create new blood vessels to feed a growing tumour. Every cell in your body gets its essentials—oxygen, nutrients, and waste removal—through a tiny blood vessel called a capillary. Every one of them! And there are about 37 trillion in the average body! As a tumour grows, the inner cells need to be served by blood vessels, not just the ones on the surface, so blood vessel growth is important and stunting this process can effectively control the growth of tumours. Cells without a blood supply die—a good thing in this case.

An excellent description of how chemo works is provided by chemo-care.com:

> Chemotherapy is most effective at killing cells that are rapidly dividing. Unfortunately, chemotherapy does not know the difference between cancer cells and normal cells. The "normal" cells will grow back and be healthy but in the meantime side effects occur. The "normal" cells most commonly affected by chemotherapy are the blood cells, the cells in the mouth, stomach and bowel, and the hair follicles resulting in low blood counts, mouth sores, nausea, diarrhea, and/or hair loss. Different drugs may affect different parts of the body (20).

Here's where fasting's superpower comes in. Throughout a human's lifespan, we have some cells that continue in active growth, even once we're fully developed. These include our hair follicles, our bone marrow, which produces blood cells of various types, our immune system and the linings of our digestive tract and airways. Once we're adults, most of the other rapid growth areas (bones, muscles, etc.) go into a maintenance phase. This involves continued repair and replacement of cells but not active growth (that's why we don't get any taller after puberty). Chemotherapy, as a blunt weapon, is sent into the body to find rapidly growing and dividing cells and will mistakenly also impact on our healthy cells that are in rapid metabolic mode. That's why hair loss, bone marrow and immune system depression, and gastrointestinal symptoms (right from the mouth to the rectum) are its common side effects.

But what if there were a way to put your healthy cells into "stealth mode?" What if we could slow down the metabolism of our healthy cells so that they become invisible to the chemo drugs? Well, there is, and we can! THAT'S FASTING'S SUPERPOWER!

As a basic survival mechanism of all lifeforms, from single-cell organisms to plants to warm-blooded mammals, such as ourselves, we all have the ability to slow down our metabolism and put ourselves into a waiting mode when our nutrient supply is threatened or cut off. If we didn't, we would never be able to fuel our full-on metabolic processes and we would run out of energy quickly. Not unlike a machine, we have safeguards in place that allow us to "power down" our metabolism, a "protected mode" where our cells can safely wait for the next infusion of fuel. As soon as the energy supply is restored—you eat something calorie-containing—then the brakes come off and the cells go back into normal metabolic function.

This is different than chronic starvation, where there's some energy but not enough. The body will try to maintain normal function but reduce the number of cells asking for fuel. Starvation—or chronic caloric restriction—leads to a loss of muscle tissue over time, as well as fat stores. Fasting does not, as the following 2016 study shows (31).

A group of obese adults was split into two groups. One group did eight weeks of alternate day fasting, eating whatever they wanted on the days in between. The second group ate a traditional calorie-restricted diet, at a 400 kcal/day deficit. Both groups lost a similar amount of weight, but the intermittent fasting group lost only 1.2 kg of lean mass (meaning muscle tissue) compared to 1.6 kg in the calorie restriction group. This indicated a sparing of protein and an increased amount of fat loss as a percentage of overall weight. Importantly, the fasting group lost more than double the amount of the more dangerous visceral (belly) fat.

The same study also proved some other important benefits of fasting. Chronic (ongoing) calorie restriction reduces basal metabolic rate, the "starvation mode" effect that doctors and dietitians have talked about for years. Eating small, inadequate meals frequently, the way we have been teaching for years, causes the body to always be circulating insulin and promoting blood sugar fluctuations (leading to hunger and cravings) and restricting the release of fats from the body's stores. Your whole metabolism will slow down in response to this chronic undernutrition. You are effectively starving your cells despite being surrounded by riches of extra stored energy. How many of us have eaten the classic "Special K breakfast" (bowl of low-fibre cereal, low-fat milk, a few berries, fruit juice) and been ravenously hungry and ready to punch someone two hours later? Cue the mid-morning low-fat cereal bar. Repeat throughout the day. The non-scientific name for this state is "hangry."

Intermittent fasting, on the other hand, was shown to not reduce the basal metabolic rate. Because fasting causes insulin levels in the blood to drop dramatically, it induces the release of counter-regulatory hormones, whereas chronic calorie restriction does not. The body is switching fuel sources, rather than shutting itself down, slowing itself down for temporary protection and switching to body-fat-derived energy—fatty acids and ketone bodies, in particular.

Another major difference is that chronic calorie restriction increases ghrelin, the hunger hormone, whereas fasting does not. That means that you experience significantly less hunger when fasting. This difference is even more pronounced if you are already following a low-carb or ketogenic diet, as you have the metabolic flexibility already built in to allow you to access and burn stored body fat for fuel.

All that to say that fasting is not only safe, it's a natural state, one that the body is fully prepared for. Our incredibly smart bodies are not only capable of surviving a fast, we thrive through it! Hormonal response to a drop in insulin during a fast allows for an increase in metabolic rate, increase in growth hormone, breakdown of damaged or duplicate protein structures, and an efficient use of our stored energy—the fat stores. It's an elegant and fascinating process.

Chemotherapy drugs, laser-focussed on rapidly metabolizing cells, will bypass most of our normal tissues when they are in the fasted state. Although exact mechanisms are still being discovered, there's evidence of this effect in everything from single-celled organisms to simple worms to mice to humans. At the same time, it's important to note that this effect of fasting doesn't protect tumour cells as well, a phenomenon that has been thoroughly investigated over the past 20 years by Dr. Longo at UCLA. (See the Additional References and Links section in the Appendix.) The difference between the "protected survival mode" of our healthy cells and the increased sensitivity of cancer cells to the chemotherapy drugs has been named the "differential stress response" (32).

In 2009, Dr. Longo published a case study report of 10 cancer patients who used fasting during chemotherapy (6). A variety of types and stages of cancer were represented. Subjects used a variety of fasting protocols and some fasted for only certain cycles, choosing to eat as desired for the other cycles. Patients reported side effects incidence and severity for each cycle. Of the subjects, four had breast cancer, two had prostate cancer, and one each had ovarian, lung, uterine, and esophageal cancers. Fasting times ranged from 48–140 hours prior to and 5–56 hours after chemo. All of the subjects experienced reduced side effects of chemotherapy. Fasting prior to and after chemotherapy treatment was concluded to be an effective intervention for reducing side effects.

When I first found and read this study, I hungrily looked for similarities between my situation and the people described in the article. I particularly resonated with Case 1, a 51-year-old woman with breast cancer who took her first chemotherapy fasted, and had minimal side effects, even returning to work shortly after. She was talked into not fasting for cycles 2 and 3 and had a much worse response: Moderate to severe fatigue, weakness, nausea, abdominal cramps, and diarrhea. These times she was forced to take additional time off work. She returned to fasting for her remaining chemo sessions and side effects again became minimal. In addition, her blood work was not as deeply depressed when she fasted, indicating that her bone marrow was being protected as well.

I also identified with Case 5, a 74-year-old woman receiving exactly the same drugs and schedule as me, in her case for uterine cancer. She ate through the first cycle and experienced significant fatigue, weakness, hair loss, headache, and gastrointestinal discomfort. From cycle 2 onward, she fasted and reported a significantly lessened severity of side effects.

This was the one article that had the most impact on my decision to use fasting as an intervention for chemo side effect management. I then worked backwards and dove into the research on lesser animals and organisms. This area of study began in 1988—it's not last-minute stuff. And it's incredibly effective but still relatively unknown. My oncologist, Dr. S, wasn't aware of fasting as an intervention, his clinic staff weren't, most of the online cancer community wasn't. I didn't ever meet the cancer centre dietitians but it's likely that they weren't aware of this intervention either.

Not everyone would be suitable for fasting around chemo cycles and not everyone is willing to make the effort. Given our cultural relationship with food, vast numbers of people are totally unaware that it's even possible to go more than a few hours without food. But it deserves to be discussed and offered as a possible approach, one that puts the power of self-determination back into the hands of the person experiencing cancer.

Animals and babies are aware that they're in control of whether they eat or not. It's one of the first areas of self-determination that we develop as infants and one of the last areas of self-awareness that the aged and even people with end-stage dementia can manage to control. Whether we open our mouths and accept food is within our own control. In the crazy vortex of treatments, specialists, tests, surgeries, and emotions that is the cancer journey, what and whether we eat is one anchoring point of self-determination. By becoming informed consumers and patients, we can manage our experience, improve our outcomes, and feel a sense of control in an often out-of-control situation. It's free—absolutely no additional expense involved. That makes fasting accessible to everyone.

It has become my passion to get the message out to others with cancer that there's a powerful way for you to be in control of one aspect of your care. The cancer establishment needs to wake up to the truth that there's a metabolic defect that is common to almost all cancers and that it can be exploited by a notion as simple as fasting and dietary choices. Research is ongoing in ketogenic diets for cancer treatment but little work has yet been done on using the combination of keto diet and fasting for impacting cancer growth, treatment effectiveness, and side effect management.

A review of the current research situation, published in 2018, was entitled, "To Fast or Not to Fast Before Chemotherapy, That Is the Question." From that article:

> Whether the results obtained by fasting in the cellular and animal models can be transferred to cancer patients is still to be ascertained. At the moment, more preclinical studies are required to determine in which cancers, at which stage, and in what combinations fasting, fasting-mimicking diets, or caloric restriction mimetics may prove effective (21).

Unfortunately, most articles review the information on fasting and calorie restriction as though they are the same thing. But as we have discussed, fasting leads to a different hormonal and metabolic response than calorie restriction and deserves to be studied as its own specific intervention. Hopefully, this work will continue and be published in coming years.

Create a Circle of Care

"In everyone's life, at some time, our inner fire goes out. It is then burst into flame by an encounter with another human being. We should all be thankful for those people who rekindle the inner spirit."
—**Albert Schweitzer**

Everybody is different in regard to how much of themselves they share with others. I have friends who would never let anyone know about what's going on in their lives and others who publish their entire physical and emotional journey on Facebook. It's a very personal decision. I think that I fall somewhere in the middle. In some situations, I will put on a brave face and enthuse that "Everything is just great!" in my life, and at other times, I'm quite willing to say, "Well, I'm struggling a bit." As a deeply optimistic person, it's hard to tell others that things suck. Even if I do say something to that effect, I generally follow it up immediately with a "Well, but…" and have a positive silver-lining type view of whatever the situation is. Cancer is like that—it sucks but there's lots of silver-lining aspects to it.

A cancer diagnosis is a pretty hard thing to hide. If your "normal" life involves a workplace, a social circle, friends and acquaintances, possibly volunteering jobs, or other activities, there's going to be a major disruption to the status quo. There's medical appointments and possible surgical interventions that are going to mean missed work or screwed up schedules. There's the very obvious physical differences of hair loss and weight changes. And there's the change in your face and your inner light that reveals to the astute observer that you're carrying a burden…

I knew from the start that I would be sharing my cancer diagnosis with my circle of family, friends, coworkers, and acquaintances. It simply wasn't a secret that I was going to be able to keep. However, I had to live with it myself for a while before I was ready to share it with others.

One of the things that I wasn't aware of until I started telling others about my diagnosis was that you need to be able to absorb their reaction into yourself. People are often devastated to hear about a diagnosis and you almost have to help *them* to process it. It takes emotional energy and strength to do this so be settled about it within yourself before you tell others.

I work in a long-term care facility with about 100 employees and 100 residents. I've been there for 14 years but only for two days a week and only as a consultant dietitian. I have never been on the payroll, in the union, or part of the lunchroom crowd. So when I knew that I was facing surgery, chemotherapy, losing my hair, and messing up my regularly sched-uled days, I wrote an open letter to the staff and posted it on the fridge door in the staff room. I clearly stated my diagnosis and upcoming path; I thanked them for their understanding and asked for support, prayers, and healing energy during my journey. Likewise, I came out on social media but only after I had told the friends who mattered in person. This was all of my family, my congregation, my best friends (the "Cottage Girls"), and my knitting group ladies.

An amazing thing happens when you reveal to the world that you have a serious medical situation, particularly the "Big C." Everyone is differently affected by the news. Some relive a loved one dealing with a similar situa-tion, perhaps dying from it. It's too painful and raw for them to be able to face the same thing in you so they distance themselves. Others simply feel like they don't know what to say so they fade away. Some don't want to deal with you if you can't be your usual self in your usual role so they retreat to await the return of the "real you."

However, for everyone that fades out of your life, there will be others, often unexpected, who will rush in. After I posted the letter on the fridge at work, I had many staff members drop by my office to offer best wishes and support. Some of them were people that I would have considered the most superficial of acquaintances, yet there they were, authentically caring about my situation enough to tell me. I had cards and food and offers of rides or other help from friends and friends of friends.

I have always been fiercely independent and I could never stand to be fussed over. Taking help from others was a muscle that I didn't use very much and I had to exercise it until I was comfortable being the receiver rather than the giver.

What I learned was that many people *want* to help, they *want* to give, they *want* to share your burden. Sometimes they simply need a bit of guidance as to how. I was gifted with prayer shawls (two of them!), a most beautiful, love-infused cuddle quilt, several bracelets, flowers, a journal, and food, lots of food! Some of the food fit into my very strict keto guidelines and some didn't, but all of it was appreciated and consumed by either Mike or me. Keeping my caregiver fed was just as big a help as giving me something that I could eat myself.

There were several times when I had to reach out to my circle of friends and supporters and do a big ask. Twice, I needed a ride to London for chemo because of Mike's immovable commitments. Friends stepped up both times and drove me down, stayed with me overnight, accompanied me to clinic appointments and chemo, then drove me home. One of those trips was a terrifying drive down through blizzard conditions followed by getting storm-stayed in southern Ontario because all the roads at home were closed. That wonderful, level-headed, unflappable friend stayed an extra night and then drove me home 24 hours later. Once we realized that the highways were all closed and we couldn't get home on schedule, I made a call to nearby friends, out of the blue, and asked another big favour—a night at their bed and breakfast with only a few hours' notice. Although they didn't even know about my cancer prior to that call, they were wonderfully gracious and accommodating, welcoming my friend and me into their home on a blustery February night.

As I have said before, and will again before this book is done, cancer is a gamechanger. It clears the cobwebs out of your life and makes it apparent what and who is important. As you travel your cancer journey, you might be surprised at who travels by your side and who doesn't. Don't judge those who make themselves scarce. You will never know what emotions are stirred up by facing cancer in another person. It's frightening to have your comfortable relationship with someone rocked off its foundation by huge physical and psychological changes. What do I say? How will my friend be different? Can I cope with their possible negativity, fear, pain? What if they die?

Know who is in your inner circle of care and who is in the broader group. The immediate inner circle folks need to know where you are at, both physically and mentally, and they should hear it from you or your most trusted caregiver. The rest can get the information by dissemination. Know who you can ask for physical favours (rides, to pick up groceries or supplies) and who is there to listen and be supportive. They will likely be different people—some are "do-ers," others are "be-ers," my made-up word for those who are simply present to listen, empathize, support, and love. Know who your "experts" are—those who have gone through a similar experience. Know who you can text in the middle of the night because they might be awake and looking at their phone.

Becoming the centre of a circle of care is one of the best outcomes from a cancer diagnosis. It allows you to realize how truly blessed you are by friends and acquaintances. It can be an uncomfortable fit at first—it certainly was for me—but I consider those growing pains to be a necessary part of my journey. Now I know that I can support and love another through the toughest times when my turn comes to be in the circle of care.

Make Social Media Work for You

I got tired of answering the heartfelt question, "How are you doing?" People would say it with the kindest, most sympathetic look on their faces, searching in my eyes for that scared, unwell cancer "victim" that they assumed lived inside my head. It was obvious from my appearance that things weren't normal—the lack of eyebrows and eyelashes was a dead giveaway. The knitted hat worn in the office at midday was a sure-fire clue...

They meant well, but I didn't want to give them what they were looking for—the type of answer that said, "It's tough, but I'm holding up okay" or "I'm fighting the good fight." I wanted them to know that I was having two awesome weeks every cycle with one not-so-awesome week in between. That I wasn't in a "battle." That I was loving my ability to manage and minimize my own symptoms. That I was actually all fired up about this new information and the strategy that I was using. That I couldn't wait to tell others so that more people with cancer could reduce their side effect burden and thus improve their quality of life as well. All of that is hard to convey in a one sentence answer.

That's where social media came in. It was a way to share my journey with a large group of people efficiently and with minimal personal interaction. Instead of having to emotionally bear the burden of those asking about me, I could put my message out in the way that was most important to me. I could add pictures of my own choosing and present the real underlying joy of what I was feeling. There were no pictures of my "nausea" face (seldom happened), no grumbling posts about how restrictive my diet was (because it wasn't), or how hard fasting was (because it wasn't). Instead, there's a snowshoeing picture, hilarious shaving-of-the-head pictures, knitting my way through chemo pictures, and lots of food pictures. And pictures of my gorgeous bald head covered in flowers and vines and paisley patterns drawn there by my Cottage Girls. On Facebook, I could share my wonderful blessings with everyone far and wide and collect the likes and comments that buoyed me up and helped me to feel even more loved.

It was also early in my chemotherapy journey that I started my blog and a new Facebook page to support the blog. I was passionately interested in sharing the information that I had learned during my research and to share the protocol that I had developed and was working so well for me. Social media allowed me to reach past my immediate circle of friends and tell my story to a wider audience.

Believe me when I say that early in my cancer process, I searched high and low for the stories of others travelling a similar path. I knew that I wanted to put my story out there for other women to find. My blog and Facebook page were my way of doing that. This book is also a part of that passion to share my story so that others can know that they are not alone and certainly not powerless in the face of cancer.

Not everyone will want to share as openly as I did. Social media is a tool and can be used judiciously to keep far-flung family and friends aware of the current situation without the need for multiple phone calls and the personal energy drain that can entail. If social media isn't part of your everyday repertoire, you could ask someone in your circle of care to be responsible for keeping the wider world aware of your situation and your progress.

Asking for support from your remote contacts can be powerful. You can request prayers, healing thoughts, distance Reiki, universal energy life force, whatever type of positive energy the person practices. Although this can sound pretty "woo-woo," there's sound evidence of a positive universal energy that we can all call on and connect to whenever we are open and ready to receive. Call it God, Holy Spirit, the Law of Attraction, the Universe, whatever resonates with your being—you know it exists and is a power for good.

A word of warning…social media is not the place to break important news to people in your inner circle. Your initial diagnosis and what that means for you is not a topic to broadcast across Facebook if you haven't yet told your spouse, your kids, your parents, or your boss. Those tough conversations need to happen face-to-face, or at least voice-to-voice over a phone call. But social media is a great place to share progress with coworkers, teammates, acquaintances, fellow volunteers, or neighbours. Then when you run into them later, the conversation will be more like this: "Hey, I saw your post about going snowshoeing. That's so cool! It's great that you have the energy for that!" Such a positive, upbeat start to a conversation.

Getting feedback on your posts can also feel like your whole community is rallying around you. Likes, comments, thumbs-ups, and shares are all so reassuring. Your message is being heard—you matter to others. I would pull up the list of all the readers who had liked my posts and read them one by one, thinking about each person who had made the effort to acknowledge them. Comments were even more treasured, as most were truly uplifting. I felt connected and supported. It was another way to feel universal love, right from the comfort of my recliner or even the chemo bed. They were cherished reminders that I mattered and that others were thinking of me or praying for me.

Connect to Spirit – Feel Blessed

"There is a LIGHT in this world. A healing spirit more powerful than any darkness we may encounter. We sometimes lose sight of this force when there is suffering, and too much pain. Then suddenly, the spirit will emerge through the lives of ordinary people who hear a call and answer in extraordinary ways."
— **Richard Attenborough**

It's easy to feel isolated when you receive a cancer diagnosis and start down the path of treatment. You're required to step out of many of the roles and responsibilities of your life, the things that define you as who you are. It's disconcerting to you but it's also very discomfiting for those around you. You might be the "co-worker" or "the athlete" or "the parent" or "the volunteer" or "the mailman." We all play a variety of roles in our everyday existence. We understand them and those around us understand them. It turns our world upside down when someone steps out of their box and into a totally new reality.

We generally aren't very good at absorbing the emotions of others without feeling their pain or fear so we put up barriers to protect ourselves. Some individuals are what's called "empaths," those who connect to others on such a visceral level that they can hardly bear to feel another's emotions. Others order their world by putting everyone they meet into predetermined "boxes" and look at everyone as a "specimen" defined by the box they're in.

Then there are the walled-off individuals who don't really let anyone into their bubble. It might be fear that keeps them locked into their own little version of reality but it's as much a prison on the inside as it is protection from the outside. These people are often sad.

One of the hardest roles for me to give up was that of the "superwoman." A strong, healthy, vibrant, look-at-me-almost-60-and-no-wrinkles superwoman. Vulnerability has never been one of my strengths. Frailty was for others, not me! I thrived and even preened when others made comments about how great I was at doing so many things at once. Like I said—superwoman…

Once I got over being knocked off that pedestal, I had to find other ways to feel my strength and blessings. I did that by connecting my inner spirit to the greater spirit—God, the Universe, Nature—however you choose to describe it. For me, that meant a rock-solid faith in a greater spirit that is universal love, always referred to in my life as God. In secular spiritualism, Universe or Universal Spirit is more commonly used. Although membership in traditional religions is shrinking, there's still a huge proportion of people who realize that we are all connected to each other and the earth by an overarching energy. It's in us and around us. As is my understanding of God. We all contain God within us and we all are beloved children of that divine energy.

Dealing with a potentially life-threatening diagnosis is a good time to realize that you are not alone and that we are all part of an interconnected web of life. Putting my vulnerability out there for all to see was hard for me but allowed connection to other kindred souls going through a similar experience. It also allowed me to attract and accept help from many caring friends and acquaintances. And it gave me the emotional resilience to accept this new wrinkle in my path and use my knowledge and skill to find ways to help myself.

I am blessed with a generations-deep heritage in a faith community. I know that the power of communal prayer lifted me though my surgeries and chemo treatments. Friends and acquaintances from all over Ontario kept me in their thoughts and prayers through that time. Now that is something that I can do to pay it forward—pray for others.

Each person will have their own relationship with the greater power that is all around and within us. If you haven't had much time to think on this, now is probably as good a time as any. Life is only richer when we connect with others—there are no downsides. Connecting with spirit might entail quiet meditation, time in nature, being creative with music or art, or simply sitting still and counting your blessings. Keeping a gratitude journal is a common practice for opening oneself to universal spirit. Every day, sit intentionally and write about what good things are in your life. Some days it might be a very small victory, such as eating a meal and keeping it down. Other days it might be a phone call from a friend. No matter how crappy your day may seem on the surface, there's always something to be thankful for. Look for it and acknowledge it.

Clear the Noise of Life...

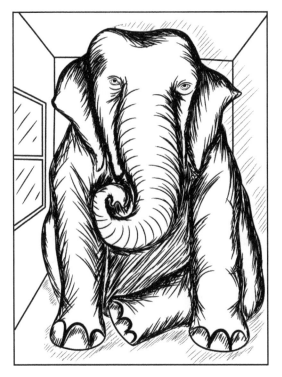

Cancer is an elephant. A freaking big elephant in the room of life. Simply receiving the diagnosis causes a huge thud in the pit of your stomach, and that's the feeling and the sound of an elephant taking up residence. From that first moment, it can't be ignored.

In early 2018, like many women of my age and stage of life, I carried many responsibilities and wore many hats. My "mom" hat was still firmly in place, despite us being empty-nesters and having two sons in their late twenties. My youngest son has a moderate developmental disability and although he has been living very successfully in his own apartment in town, he still requires intensive daily interaction, often in the form of up to eight phone calls per day. If he has become anxious or upset by something, he might need to be talked off of a figurative ledge. He frequently needs help to see all sides of a decision before he can confidently step forward in one direction or another. I still take him grocery shopping twice monthly, and most of his other shopping is done with Mom along to help him make good choices. I am his financial decision-maker and all-around cheerleader in life.

Another hat I wore was that of ordained minister and pastor to my little congregation in my hometown. Although it's a lay ministry position (not a regular job, and unpaid), it involved being part of most decisions, chairing most priesthood and business meetings, and always being available at the end of an email or a phone call. And it meant being the first one at church to unlock the doors, turn on the lights, and power up the sound system; making sure that the music works, setting up tables for potluck, making coffee for small group ministry, and taking communion to shut-ins most months. It was also a mental responsibility that was just as wearying as the physical responsibility.

Workwise, I was self-employed with contracts to provide Registered Dietitian services at three long-term care facilities, all of them requiring a specified number of hours per month. Juggling the schedules of the three homes was often challenging. In addition, I had just opened my private practice, Primal RD, to follow my passion into teaching Low Carb Healthy Fats (LCHF) living to help with healthy aging, type 2 diabetes, metabolic syndrome, and a variety of other inflammatory-based conditions.

In my "spare" time, I volunteered alongside Mike with the Little Theatre and had accepted the position of wardrobe lead on a play being put on in the fall. It was a huge job that I was really not fully qualified for—or capable of. I'm a great organizer but do not have the "artistic vision" to create a wardrobe from scratch. I felt like I was in over my head…

Add into that mix my own interests, such as being the chief organizer for the KnitWits, my small group of knitting ladies that met every Wednesday evening at church. I was responsible for opening up, locking up, making cancellation decisions based on the weather, social activities, and any member issues.

After my diagnosis, I first had to come to terms with the fact that I was now a "person with cancer." That was necessary before I could start to tell others. But gradually, I was able to see my "elephant" and understand that if it was going to settle into my life for the next few months, I needed to make room. What about all the responsibilities I carried? Who would make sure that the church sound system was turned on before service? Who would open the building for KnitWits and make sure the chairs were arranged? Who would take communion to our senior members in long-term care if not me?

In the end, I made enough room in my life for the elephant. I know that it won't take up so much space in the long term but during active diagnosis, treatment, and follow-up, it consumed enormous amounts of both physical time and emotional space. It's hard to step out of roles where you feel important, needed, essential. But the world is a big place and it won't stop spinning just because you have to step off the ride for a while.

I have found that, with time, the elephant has shrunk and will eventually be reduced to an ornament to be displayed on a shelf in my "life room." It will always be there, part of what I have gone through, but will no longer be a major disruptor. Simply one of the mementos of a life well lived.

Avoiding "You Poor Dear" Syndrome

"If you are always trying to be normal, you will never know how amazing you can be."
— **Maya Angelou**

You know the look—the "poor you" look that so many acquaintances will adopt when they address you. It's well-meaning, but sometimes you just don't want to be reminded that you have cancer or that you are going through treatment. Yes, I am aware that I don't look like myself. Yes, I am aware that I look God-awful without eyelashes or eyebrows. Yes, I am wearing a knitted cap at work. So what?

I refused to assume a victim mentality for many of the reasons described in the previous chapters of this book. Despite how I looked, I could feel power surging through me most days. My "bad days" were really just the occasional "bad spells," and I wanted everyone to know how freaking awesome I was doing, in spite of the surgeries and the chemo. I didn't want pity or well-meaning but misinformed advice, but I was always open to hear someone else's story about their or a loved one's cancer experience. I was grateful for offers of help, gifts of food, prayers, and healing thoughts. But pity? No thanks!

In the middle of treatment, my husband and I attended a concert presented by a very gifted theatre friend where I knew there'd be dozens of people there who knew us. I had found a really funky hobo-chic type dress and wore it with tall black boots, some drawn-on eyebrows, and a black and white headscarf. I felt like a million bucks, despite being bald with no eyebrows. I got lots of compliments and no pity. I expect it was because of the energy I put out that night—vibrant, alive, truly happy.

Another time, I had my three best friends in the world come to my house for a weekend visit while hubby was away. It was near the end of my fourth chemo cycle and I was feeling a bit run down but relatively well. As a fun, life-affirming gift to me, my girlfriends got "tattoo markers" and spent an afternoon drawing gorgeous multicoloured flowers and shapes onto my bald head. They didn't last for much more than a day but we captured the fun in pictures. I felt beautiful and so loved.

How others see you is very much under your control. Exude positivity, be happy and full of gratitude, see the silver lining in every situation (even if you feel crappy). It's hard to pity someone who approaches life like that. In fact, you become a blessing to others when you glow with the inner strength and energy of your convictions. You are freaking STRONG to be going through the cancer experience—that's your superpower!

Caring for Your Caregiver

"It's not how much you do, but how much love you put into the doing."
—**Mother Teresa**

Cancer is not a team sport but it sure requires a team to manage it. As the person going through cancer, it can seem to be a very solitary pursuit. Only *you* are being cut into, poked with countless needles, being radiated like a bag of microwave popcorn, or filled with toxic chemicals. Only *you* get the joys of nausea, debilitating fatigue, constipation, and baldness.

But make no mistake. Cancer takes its toll on everyone that you come in contact with. And at the top of that list is your primary caregiver. It might be a spouse or significant other, it might be a parent, a sibling, or an adult child. It might even be a young child, like me when my mother died of breast cancer—I was 18. I wasn't the primary caregiver—my dad was—but my younger brother and I were too close to not be deeply affected.

It hurts to watch someone you love as they suffer. It causes heart pain to be powerless in the face of another's hurt. It's wrenching to have to inflict further suffering on a loved one, even if it's as simple as driving them to chemo or repositioning them in bed.

It's also hard for a lover to watch their beloved change physically as baldness, bloating, weight loss or gain, incontinence, surgical scars, or radiation burns change them from who they used to be. It's even more terrifying to see someone become a stranger as possible depression, chronic pain, or brain metastases change their personality. Formerly positive, upbeat, lively people can become morose, grumpy, irritable, or even irrational.

It also hurts to feel like your future with your loved one is being threatened. It can be threatened by a shortened timeframe, a lack of certainty of growing old together. It can be threatened by a different physical reality if the cancer leaves the patient with permanent disabilities. It can even threaten one's financial future, although that's not as much of an issue in countries with socialized medical care. However, if you are interested in pursuing alternative treatments outside of the conventional path, you're likely to be funding that pursuit yourself, possibly decimating your savings. Certainly, a cancer diagnosis generally results in lost work time or reduced ability to manage job responsibilities. For those without a full-time job and sick benefits, that can be difficult.

The caregiver is sometimes forgotten in all the hoopla around the cancer patient themselves. In fact, they generally remain nameless in the whole medical system. In all the years of dealing with my developmentally challenged son and his seizure disorder, I was always just "Mom." I never had my own name. I noticed the same thing happening to my husband as we traversed the cancer care system. I will be forever grateful to my oncologist, Dr. S, for remembering Mike's name and asking him how his latest theatre production was coming along. He remembered that detail from our initial conference and referred to it in subsequent visits.

Being the caregiver can be a thankless job and yet it is deserving of so much thanks. The caregiver, naturally, experiences their own fear, grief, and uncertainty but none of this is generally acknowledged.

My primary caregiver, my husband Mike, stepped into the role of supporter, backer, driver, rationalizer, cool head, and coffee fetcher. It was hard for me not to always be the one in control. I continued to do all of the meal planning and prep, as this was something that really mattered to me and it was where I chose to put my energy. Often meal prep was simply bacon and eggs, followed by crawling into my recliner again, but it was mine to control. Mike was great at stepping back when I wanted to do something myself (not hovering or shushing me back into submission) but stepping in immediately if I needed help or had to leave a job in mid-stream. It was a fine line but he danced it well.

Caregivers need tending and watering and loving just as much as the person with cancer. I was careful to include Mike in every conversation with those calling to check in on me. And to acknowledge him and his support at every turn. I called him "my rock."

Tips for caring for your caregiver:

- Be eternally grateful. Saying "thanks" goes a long way but can get forgotten in the fog of pain, drugs, or depression.
- Acknowledge your caregiver's concerns and fears. Reassure them that you are still *you*, that you love them and so appreciate their strength in your time of weakness.
- Give your caregiver praise and show gratitude in front of others. It reminds your visitors that they need to be acknowledged and included in their caring concern.
- Do what you can for yourself. Don't take your caregiver for granted or abuse their willingness to help. While Mike was willing to drive into town at 11:00 p.m. on a cold stormy night to get me needed medication, I certainly wouldn't send him on that kind of an errand because I felt like pizza.
- Continue to contribute to the household as much as you can. Fold laundry, empty the dishwasher, make your bed every morning. Be as slow as you need to. Just don't develop a sense of entitlement— you are not a princess. You are a partner.
- Have a smile every time your caregiver looks at you. Even if you are smiling through your pain. That eye-to-eye connection is so important and reassuring for both of you.
- When you feel well—between treatments or after they're over— plan to do something very special with your loved one. It could be a special event or meal out or a weekend getaway. It could be as simple as shopping together for a new piece of furniture for your shared space or a piece of art. We went snowshoeing, very slowly…
- Always remember that the tables could turn at some time in the future and you could be caring for your lover. Be aware of the preciousness of life and health and connection.
- Gratitude, gratitude, gratitude. Life is precious.

The Universe Has Your Back

"Trust that your wounds are exactly as the Universe planned. They were divinely placed in your life in the perfect order so that you could show up for them with love and remember the light within."
— **Gabrielle Bernstein,** *The Universe Has Your Back: Transform Fear to Faith*

I saw the movie *The Secret* many years ago. I can also distinctly remember watching *What the Bleep Do We Know?* Both movies are based on the premise that our perceptions create our reality and that we are part of everything around us. The only separation from others and the Universe is one that we create ourselves from our own inner turmoil.

The idea of the glass half empty versus the glass half full is a visual representation of this idea. How we perceive that partially full glass is coloured by our paradigm—the mental, spiritual, and emotional place from which we look out at the world. Two people can look at the same object or the same situation and see totally different things and hence react in totally different ways.

Here's an example: As I write this, there's a veritable blizzard going on outside. High winds, moderate to heavy snow, drifts piling up, roads being closed. All kinds of businesses closed their doors early and events and meetings have been cancelled. It's supposed to last all night and into tomorrow.

For some people, looking out on the "ravages of nature" will fill them with depression and despondency. Damn winter! Now I have to blow the driveway, clean off my car, wear my warmest hat, and my fingers are going to freeze because I forgot to get gas for the car. My yoga class was cancelled. I ran out of milk. I'm housebound and bored...

Others will look out on the winter wonderland and marvel at the sharp, perfect crests on the drifts across their yards. They will consider it a contest to see how wild the blowing snow can get—bragging rights when you can't even see to the road in front of the house. They will welcome the opportunity for the unexpected free time that being storm-stayed affords them and will plan for a satisfying activity such as baking or crafting or reading a long-awaited book. They will be thankful that they are home safe from the storm and that the electricity hasn't gone out.

Same situation, different perceptions. Positivity vs. negativity. Glass half full vs. glass half empty.

In *What the Bleep Do We Know?* we're introduced to the idea that reality is only what we perceive, and that we can change what we perceive by being aligned with positivity and the positive energy of the Universe. *The Secret's* premise is that there is a universal Law of Attraction that each person invites into themselves whatever they're thinking about, whether good or bad. We used to call that luck...

In her book, *The Universe Has Your Back*, Gabrielle Bernstein combines these ideas by suggesting that when you are filled with love for yourself and others and when you are truly grateful for your situation, then wonderful things will come into your life and experience. Even things that seem hard or challenging or hurtful have a reason for being and that if you can approach them from a position of love, you will see why they are there and be open to learning from them. She refers to the Universe as an all-encompassing energy of love that includes all life. It is our birthright to be connected to this energy, but the sad fact is that many of us have built walls against it with our life experiences and our attitudes.

Ever since being exposed to these rather mind-blowing ideas, I have looked for the Universe in my life. I feel like many "coincidences" and "opportunities" come my way as I look for them with expectancy and positive energy. Many times, I have set an intention for something to happen or some object I need to cross my path and lo and behold, it will.

It's all pretty "woo-woo" for a rational, left-brain-dominant science geek like me and also pretty out there for a middle-aged lady raised in the Christian faith and taught to believe in a loving God. But it's really not so far from how I was raised. It was framed in the language of the church but the meanings were similar. Asking in a prayer was "setting an intention," an answer to prayer was a "blessing" or a "coincidence." The overarching love of God that is in each of our hearts is simply another explanation for the love of the Universe as described by the New-Age gurus.

When cancer happened, I had to look pretty hard for the positive side of the experience. Being handed that diagnosis was definitely a blow—physically, emotionally, and spiritually.

I didn't say, "Why did this happen to me? What did I do to deserve this? Is this going to go well, or am I starting down the path of chronic illness and premature death?" I didn't get angry or resentful.

I was scared, for sure, and bewildered. But instead, I asked myself, "What is the Universe trying to teach me with this situation? What can I do to get through this? What do I need?" And then the Universe started to deliver. It was amazing!

A friend who had recently gone through breast cancer treatment (surgery, chemo, and radiation) had given me a glowing review of her gynecological oncologist. Well, out of all the doctors at London Regional Cancer Centre, I ended up referred to him! Then it turned out that he was from my hometown and we had both been involved in high school drama productions, albeit at different schools and a couple of years apart. He had even been at the same regional drama festival as me back in the late '70s. His mother was the head dietitian at the hospital across the street from my childhood home. So many connections—it was magical!

After the very uncomfortable recovery from my first surgery, I had decided that I needed a recliner chair before going into my second, larger surgery and the months of chemotherapy ahead. Since I had never owned a recliner before, I did some research and visited several stores to try and figure out the best option. I knew that I wanted something that looked as little like a recliner as possible, not too big and puffy, a wall-hugger, and one that was electric. I didn't have bags of money to spend on the chair of my dreams either. And time was short—the next surgery was only a couple of weeks away. I couldn't order anything that would take months to be manufactured and delivered. I needed a store model or in-stock item.

I had found a reasonably good candidate at a local furniture store for about $700 but was going to check one more store in a town about an hour away. One Saturday afternoon, I set out for the drive to this far-off store. As I drove, I was actively thinking about attracting and finding my ideal chair. It would be a decent colour in a wall-hugger style that would not be ugly in my living room (brown was out!), electric, not too oversized. I was clearly setting an intention.

I had to pass the Habitat for Humanity ReStore on my way to my destination so I dropped in. All down one wall were used recliners, probably a dozen. All oversized and ugly and worn and many even brown—yuck. I wandered the whole store and was just heading toward the exit when I spotted two chairs sitting off in a whole separate area. Turns out they were over in the other corner because they needed to be plugged in! There was my chair—in a clean, grey fabric and in pristine shape, perfectly functional, and only $250—with no taxes! It had only been put on the display floor a couple of hours prior. I bought it on the spot, had them load it into the back of my car (thank goodness for SUVs), and drove it straight home. Back in 45 minutes from what was supposed to be a three-hour trip, with the perfect chair and for a fraction of the expected cost.

I firmly believe that that exact chair was put into that exact place at that exact time for me to find and claim. It's just one example of many that show me, again and again, the power of intention and the benevolence of the Universe when we are open to its loving energy.

I think about the fact that cancer appeared in my life right at this particular moment in my development as a low-carb dietitian. My knowledge of the ketogenic diet and my confidence in the power of low-carb strategies were at their strongest. If I had faced cancer even five years prior, I would not have had the confidence to use these interventions. The research around cancer metabolism has exploded in the last five years so I wouldn't have even found references to much of what I learned. The Universe brought cancer into my life exactly when I had all of the tools to deal with it.

My cancer journey has brought me here, to this place. I am writing this book to share the power of nutritional interventions to impact on wellness, healing, and cancer treatment side effects. These interventions have the power to prevent cancer development, to slow cancer growth and proliferation, and to improve overall wellness while going through treatment. Prior to getting cancer, I had no idea that any of this existed. Despite spending my entire career in dietetics, I don't think I really had any idea of the true potential power of what we eat. And if a dietitian didn't get it, how is everyone else supposed to know?

Like the quote says at the beginning of this section, our wounds—the challenges, roadblocks, setbacks, and pain—can be a gift from the Universe that sets us on a new path. "They were divinely placed in your life in the perfect order so that you could show up for them with love and remember the light within."

The timing of the wounds, and the nature of them, are gifts and opportunities if we can see them in the light of love and lean into the experience with an open heart and mind.

Keep Moving, Even Slowly

How much you exercise during cancer treatment really depends on how much you exercised prior to cancer treatment. Certainly, the middle of treatment is not the time to take on training for a marathon or a CrossFit competition, no matter your previous fitness level. The energy, both physical and mental, of dealing with cancer and cancer treatment is draining. You need to conserve that energy for your overall health, not an exercise goal.

Many people, once faced with a cancer diagnosis, will figure that there's no place for any sort of physical activity in their immediate futures and take to their (aptly named) La-Z-Boy chairs, assuming the role of invalid from the get-go. This is just about the worst thing you can do, both physically and mentally. Giving up on physical strength is just plain stupid at a time when you need to feel the power of your own body to heal itself and be the epitome of strength. Using physical exercise to support mental health is an evidence-based intervention. Exercise improves mental health by reducing anxiety, depression, and negative mood and by improving self-esteem and cognitive function (22, 23, 24). At the time of writing, there are studies underway to examine the role of exercise in women with ovarian cancer during and after chemotherapy. The results will be interesting but are probably years away yet (29).

If you were mostly sedentary prior to getting cancer, aim for gentle walks as your exercise of choice. Try to get outside every day for this exercise, no matter the time of year. Fresh moist outside air and natural light is vitally important for wellness and spiritual peacefulness. If at all possible, take off your shoes and connect directly with the ground, ideally on grass or a dirt garden path. This is a practice called "grounding" and is based on the principle that we have always, throughout evolution, been connected to the magnetic signals from the earth. Our modern life, with cars, indoor living, and shoes, has almost totally disconnected us from this very primal relationship with the earth. The Chinese have always known about "qi" or "chi" (referred to in India as "prana"). Similarly, the Earthing movement (those who practice grounding) believes that connecting to the ground allows movement of negative electrons through our bodies, reducing inflammation, calming our brains of anxiety, and improving blood flow. Modern technology allows us to measure electron fields and magnetism arising from our own bodies and from the earth. When we connect with nature we share in this planetary energy. This all sounds very "woo-woo" but we can all acknowledge that in our modern-day way of life we're living in a very disconnected way from nature.

Walking, preferably outside, is the best exercise when in the midst of cancer treatment, whether post-surgery or during chemo or radiation. It's the easiest exercise to scale up or down based on your exercise tolerance each day. Even a gentle tour of your back yard to check out the state of the garden is beneficial. On another day, when energy levels are better, aim for a longer walk at a brisker pace.

If you were much more physically active before cancer, you might be able to manage more exercise during chemo, but don't expect to maintain your previous levels of achievement. If going to the gym is good for your mental state and your fighting spirit, by all means go. But don't expect to make gains and don't even expect to maintain your current stamina. Your metabolic energy and your mental energy are going towards something much more important right now—eradicating cancer in your body. Continue going to the gym if it feeds your soul but if not, try to do gentle exercises like walking, stretching, or yoga when your energy allows.

Even in the worst days of my post-chemo funk, I would get out of my recliner every hour or so and "putz." This might take the form of emptying the dishwasher or switching the laundry into the dryer. It might mean getting into my coat and boots and walking down to the end of my driveway for the mail. If I was feeling okay, I would extend that walk a couple of hundred feet to the end of my little street. Another time I might water the plants or do some food prep for the next meal. Then when I tired out, I would happily climb back into my nest, feeling like I had accomplished something. I credit my nutritional strategies with feeling good enough to manage this level of activity, even on the "worst" days. I never had "horizontal" days. I hope that you experience the same positive results.

Pay It Forward — The Way Past Cancer

"The best way to predict the future is to create it."
—Abraham Lincoln

I have loved the concept of "pay it forward" ever since I first heard it. It's the idea that, when you've been the beneficiary of some kind of good deed or good fortune, or a gift, you don't need to pay the giver back as much as you need to become a blessing to someone else by continuing the gift forward. Often you might need to do both, especially in the case of financial or physical gifts. But many times, those in our circle of care have no ulterior motives other than love and caring for giving us the gift of their time, or perhaps a meal, or a small memento or inspirational gift. Friends arriving on my doorstep the morning after chemo with a half dozen freshly baked muffins or the neighbour who walked his snowblower over and took care of my driveway for me—these are the little kindnesses and gifts that meant so much during my chemotherapy treatment. My fellow backyard chicken rancher who shared her eggs with me while I was on chicken sabbatical. The unexpected box in the mail containing a gorgeous lap quilt from my oldest friend. These are just a few of the many blessings that I was recipient of during my chemo winter.

As you have read, I'm a big believer that the Universe (or God, omnipotent spirit—however you understand it) is a positive force for good that we can all tap into by opening ourselves spiritually to its eternal love. I'm an unrepentant optimist and I can find a silver lining in just about any situation. I also believe in meditation, prayer, and focussed intention as powerful interventions for good. I was the receiver of much of that type of loving energy from the first moment of diagnosis and throughout my cancer journey, these gifts of love and kindness are still continuing on to this day.

So when the active part of the cancer journey comes to an end, what then? Chemotherapy is over, the chemo port has been removed from my chest wall, my hair is starting to grow back in, and it's finally time to look up and around. Some of the roles and responsibilities that I gave up during my journey are starting to crowd back into my space. Do I let them in? What have I learned along the way? How am I different?

Coming back to my life after cancer was more of an adjustment than I had anticipated. At the end of the nine months of surgery and chemotherapy, there were several people waiting to give back to me the responsibilities that they had willingly shouldered in my absence. The man who had been pastor to my congregation was ready to return to his own church. The dietitian who had assumed two of my contracted nursing homes was planning how to proceed into the summer. The Little Theatre came calling, wondering if I wanted to be involved in the fall musical. I had already ordered my new chickens, ready to take on the responsibility of backyard farming again.

If I'm fully honest, I can say that I totally enjoyed having none of those responsibilities for a period of months, cancer or no cancer. And it was almost an irritation to have to pick them up again. It made me realize how many hats I wear in an average week and how many people rely on me. The roles that I never abandoned for cancer treatment—parent to my special-needs son, wife and household manager, dietitian at one long-term care facility—those were still there, but now all the nooks and crannies of my free space were going to be refilled with new (but old) responsibilities.

Coming back into my life after cancer was an opportunity to review whether I still wanted to wear all those hats. Or to what extent. Or for how much longer. I feel deeply in my bones that I am cleared of cancer and that I will now continue to live and love life for decades. But niggling in the very back recesses of my brain are the "What ifs?" What if the cancer recurs? What if it spreads? What if I don't live to a ripe old age?

Of course, we'll never know the future. We only have the present. And that makes the present pretty darn important. If it ever came down to quality over quantity, would I be satisfied with the quality of how I have lived these months and years?

So I live in the present. I look for opportunities to be happily engaged in my life, giving of my energy, my optimism, sharing my faith in the goodness of the Universe, and paying it forward with the writing of this book.

I continue to practice a whole-foods, low-carb, healthy-fats lifestyle. Most days, I skirt around the edges of ketosis. I care about the quality of the foods I eat, so I enjoy buying from local farmers and small local vendors. I plan my meals and stock my house with only healthy fats, quality meats, and lots of fresh veggies to make that easy and interesting. I am more flexible with eating out and visiting with friends, but that doesn't mean that I allow crap foods back into my space. Although I will admit to the occasional small bowl of premium potato chips (my husband's favourite indulgence), I do not allow nonorganic grains into my home and we seldom have anything containing large quantities of sugar. I practice intermittent fasting but on a rather spontaneous schedule. My food environment is organized so that I can live in the present and make decisions based on the now.

The message that we can each control our own response to cancer treatment is one that needs to get out to the wider world. Although it will take years for scientific studies to validate exact protocols, we can do things now that have little to no risk and potentially huge positive rewards. Supporting others through their cancer treatment journey is going to be my "paying it forward" for the foreseeable future. I hope that it will be a bend in my career path that truly fulfills my passion for life and for giving.

Each cancer journeyer will have their own path. Each will have to give up on certain responsibilities and dreams when cancer enters their room and takes up residence as the elephant in the corner. But along the path, there will be times when they need to decide whether to pick up the threads of their previous life. It's a time for inner examination and personal reflection. And as the elephant shrinks and takes up less space, there will be opportunities to give back or give forward.

Remember that you will now be an expert in a life experience that usually sneaks up and surprises most people. Just being able to offer reassurance that "you will get through this" will be your new superpower. Offering to accompany friends to appointments, look after pets or kids while they are sick, make them food, or weed their gardens. So many opportunities to give back.

The positive love and energy of the Universe comes to those who are open and willing to receive, then flows out to others. Put into different words: God loves you unconditionally and when you open your heart to Him, you will feel that love and it will flow through you to others. The meaning is the same.

Part 3
Practical Implementation

When Keto and Fasting Are NOT Right for You

A ketogenic diet and therapeutic fasting are powerful interventions and have major impacts on your body and your brain. Like any powerful thing, care must be taken that they are used appropriately and by those who will be helped by them, not harmed.

There are some people for whom keto and fasting are not right and some circumstances when using these dietary strategies are not recommended. Check out the list here:

1. You already have advanced cachexia. This is the official name for the severe weight loss and muscle wasting that can accompany advanced cancer. Cachexia is caused by the presence of the cancer itself and is not generally considered to be due entirely to poor nutritional intake. The pathophysiology is driven by a variable combination of nutritional intake issues and metabolic abnormalities. Many cancers and their treatments cause poor intake, leading to starvation. But in the situation of cancer cachexia, the body also appears both unable to access the nutrients taken in and to use them to maintain muscle and fat tissue in a normal manner. The underlying causes and mechanisms of cancer cachexia are still being discovered. Cachexia is a serious situation and up to 40% of cancer deaths are attributed to the presence of cachexia (30).

   Cachexia patients are at risk of a potentially serious condition called "refeeding syndrome" if they are overfed suddenly after a period of little to no calories. It is precipitated by a sudden intake of glucose (any sugary or starchy food that suddenly spikes the blood glucose) causing a corresponding sudden release of insulin and all the subsequent metabolic changes. If the body has been deprived of electrolytes (potassium, phosphorus, magnesium, or sodium) during the starvation period, there can be a sudden shift of electrolytes within the body, leading to severe organ malfunction and even death.

The type of supported three-day fast suggested in this book is not long enough or severe enough to put most people at risk of refeeding syndrome. Using bone broth and ensuring enough salt intake will minimize risk. Restarting your eating after a fast with low-carbohydrate foods will prevent the sudden rise in glucose that triggers the insulin cascade.

If you are dealing with cachexia, eating a relatively clean diet that does not include highly processed "food-like substances" will likely help greatly in nourishing your body within the limited tolerance of what you can manage. This means avoiding high-sugar foods, processed "CRAP" foods (**C**arbonated drinks, **R**efined sugar, **A**rtificial colours and flavours, and **P**rocessed products) that contain highly modified starches from industrial crops (corn, soy, wheat) and especially industrially manufactured seed oils (corn, soy, canola, sunflower), as all of these "foods" are devoid of real nutrients such as minerals, vitamins, and essential proteins and fatty acids. Even in cachexia, empty calories are not what your body needs.

2. You have a history of a diagnosed eating disorder. Fasting and severe dietary restrictions are not appropriate for anyone who has struggled with an overly restrictive relationship with food in the past. In that situation, again, eating a clean diet of unprocessed real foods in appropriate quantities is likely the best approach.

3. There is some research to suggest, in mouse models at least, that certain types of renal cell (kidney) cancers and some varieties of melanoma do not respond to a ketogenic diet in the same manner as most solid tumours (25). The evidence is very sketchy and confusing and much more needs to be done before a ketogenic diet can be recommended in this situation. Again, eating "clean"

by choosing real, unprocessed foods and avoiding ultra-processed CRAP foods is still an important approach to overall wellness.

4. If you are on insulin or blood-sugar-lowering agents for diabetes, you need to approach a keto diet carefully and with the support of your doctor or pharmacist to help with dosage adjustments. Many oral diabetic drugs work by encouraging additional insulin secretion from your own pancreas and can lead to a low blood sugar reaction when you restrict carbohydrate intake. Similarly, medications for hypertension (high blood pressure) will need to be adjusted early in the process of moving to low carb to prevent a low blood pressure situation. The need to adjust dosages of medications happens very early in the process, within days to weeks. Respect the power of the diet and the power of your medication.

The Chemo Cycle Fasting Protocol

There are no hard and fast rules around chemo fasting yet. There's much more research to be done before this will be an evidence-based protocol. But anecdotal experience documented in case studies and case series appears to favour two to three days of pretreatment fasting, enough to downregulate normal healthy cellular function, followed by 24 hours of post-chemo fasting, to keep those healthy cells quiet until the immediate chemo effect is past. This is the protocol that I followed with good results. Each person will have their own response to chemo and their cancer but this is a good place to start.

The first assumption in this protocol is that you are already following a high-fat ketogenic diet. This isn't absolutely necessary but makes the process much easier since you have the metabolic framework already in place to burn fatty acids and ketones for energy. Of course, a well-formulated, whole-foods-based ketogenic diet also protects you between chemo treatments by minimizing circulating insulin and growth factors and keeping blood sugar levels low and stable—and thus stressing cancer cells, as we have discussed already. So in preparation for your first chemo treatment, try and adopt a ketogenic diet and get your metabolic machinery in place. Ideally, three to four weeks of working towards a ketogenic diet, as described in Part 1, will put your body in a good metabolic place to undertake the fasting period. If you don't have the luxury of this time, start where you are with removing the high carb foods and processed fats from your diet, then move forward from there. Fasting will be more uncomfortable without the metabolic machinery in place to burn fats but it's not impossible. Rest assured that even if you do your first fast around a chemo treatment right from the SAD diet, you can transition out of your fast into a healthier low-carb diet and by the time the next chemo treatment comes around, you will be in a much better metabolic place.

FOR INTERMITTENT CHEMOTHERAPY—EVERY THREE WEEKS OR EVERY TWO WEEKS:

Measure out 36 hours pre-chemo. For example, if your chemo starts on a Thursday morning, count backwards: 36 hours earlier is Tuesday evening.

Measure out 24–30 hours after your chemo. If your chemo ends on Thursday afternoon, count forwards: 24–30 hours later is Friday supper-time or evening.

This is your fasting period. For a Thursday chemo, stop eating after supper on Tuesday and start again at supper on Friday. Adjust according to your chemo schedule.

PREPARATION:

Have available a minimum of 500–750 ml (2–3 cups) of bone broth. Make your own if at all possible or ask one of your support people to make it for you. Defrost it if necessary so it's ready to go.

Plan how to have coffee, tea, water, soda water, and/or bone broth available and with you at all times. Get a hold of water bottles, thermal cups, thermos flasks. Have one dedicated to only coffee as it ends up smelling of coffee and isn't much good for anything else.

Day 1: Finish eating a satisfying supper on the evening of Day 1, then consume no additional solid food or calorie-containing beverages after that. Black, green, or herbal tea, water, or soda water is fine.

Day 2: Fill your day with black coffee (with up to 1 teaspoon of heavy cream if absolutely necessary—measure it!), black, green or herbal tea, water, or soda water. It's much easier if you keep busy. Stay out of the kitchen, even out of the house if you can.

Use bone broth as a meal replacer for lunch and supper. Hot salty bone broth feels like a meal and will make your stomach feel fed.

Hunger comes in waves and then subsides. If you feel overwhelmed by hunger sensations, use additional bone broth with salt to ride it out.

Day 3: Chemo day. Continue with allowed fluids, making sure that you've made a clear plan for having your preferred fluids with you throughout your chemo visit in various thermos bottles and cups. Have your support person refill them for you as necessary. There'll usually be a coffee shop handy for tea or coffee. Drink lots of water. Avoid drinking bone broth at clinic in case of mild nausea. You don't want to associate your broth with feeling bad. If nausea becomes an issue, stick with water or water with a bit of real lemon juice.

Day 4: First day post chemo. Continue with allowed fluids, using bone broth if desired to replace lunch. Plan for a modest supper that really appeals to you. Avoid highly spicy or fatty foods for this first meal. Keto-compliant soup or scrambled eggs are light options. Don't be surprised if your appetite is pretty low despite having not eaten for three days.

KEY THINGS TO REMEMBER:

Get enough fluids. Drink, drink, drink.

Get enough salt. Use a good salt such as Himalayan pink salt or Celtic Sea salt, something with a variety of minerals present (usually as non-white flecks in the salt).

You will lose weight during the three-day fast and possibly the next day after but it's mostly water weight. Most of it will return gradually over the next week. Don't get excited or distressed by a 5–8 lb weight loss and regain. Ideally, you will only lose 1–2 lbs of actual weight per cycle at a maximum. The middle of chemotherapy is not the time to be worrying about weight loss for cosmetic purposes.

Constipation is a real risk during chemo and fasting. The combination of no digestive tract contents and the medications for chemo and side effect management can be hard on your bowel. See below for constipation protocol during chemo fasting.

What About Radiation?

Can you eat a keto diet while taking radiation treatments? What about fasting? How do you fit fasting in when radiation happens every day? How the heck does radiotherapy work anyways?

There are researchers and clinicians around the world studying and using radiation in the context of a ketogenic diet. And the results of their work, while preliminary, are all positive.

Radiation therapy works by damaging the genetic material of the cancer cells, making it impossible for the cell to divide and grow. It also leads to cell death so tumours not only don't grow well, they actually shrink. Healthy cells are better at repairing genetic damage and healing than are cancer cells. Radiotherapy is highly focussed but it can still cause collateral damage to surrounding healthy cells and that limits its use. The main side effects are nausea and bone-deep fatigue that isn't relieved by rest. Longer term, there can be radiation burn damage of nearby tissues. This can be a big problem with the digestive tract—esophagus damage in lung cancer radiation, bowel damage in pelvic cancer radiation, swallowing function damage after head or neck cancer radiation.

The ketogenic diet is being investigated as an adjunct therapy with radiation therapy to reduce inflammatory processes and to protect brain cells in brain cancers. There are fascinating studies in mouse models that show a more than cumulatively positive effect of a ketogenic diet and radiation together. In fact, in the study quoted below, most of the test mice who were fed a strict 4:1 ketogenic diet (four parts fat calories to one part protein/carb calories) and given radiation showed total remission of their implanted brain cancers. These animals went on to return to their normal diets and lived for months afterwards with no cancer—amazing! Lifespan returned to normal, despite having been intentionally implanted with brain tumours.

From the peer-reviewed and published article about their work, Dr. Adrienne Scheck and colleagues write:

> "We therefore tested KC (KetoCal—the 4:1 keto diet replacer) in addition to radiation to determine if the effect of the two treatments would be more than additive. *Nine out of the 11 animals treated with KC in combination with radiation were apparently cured of their implanted tumour.* (emphasis added)
>
> "In conclusion, we demonstrated that the effect of a ketogenic diet was more than additive when used in combination with radiation for the treatment of glioma in a mouse model system" (26).

Most of the work done so far in this area has concentrated on brain tumours, as it is already known in cases of epilepsy that ketones in the blood will be used by the brain as an alternate fuel with good results. There appears to be little to no risk and considerable potential benefit from using a ketone-producing diet and further research will eventually branch out past brain tumours to include other commonly irradiated cancers, such as breast cancer and colon cancer.

Because the treatment schedule for radiation generally involves five consecutive daily treatments over a period of four to six weeks, there is no role for extended fasting. However, maintaining ketosis using a restricted diet and possible intermittent fasting may be beneficial. Intermittent fasting refers to the practice of restricting the eating period of each day to a short, defined time span, with the remainder of the day in a fasted state. Many people follow a pattern of 16 hours fasted and an eating "window" of eight hours. This could be used for radiation therapy by planning your fasts and eating around the time of your treatment. For example, if the daily treatment is at 11:00 a.m., you would finish supper by 7:00 p.m. and then not eat again until after radiation, perhaps at noon the following day. That would provide a 16-hour fast prior to the radiation "pulse," putting your body further into ketosis in preparation. Meal intake would be lunch, possibly an afternoon snack, then supper. Then fast again after supper until the next day's treatment is done.

If your treatment is in late afternoon, you might eat a very low-carb, possibly zero-carb breakfast, then fast through lunch until after the treatment, then enjoy a dinner and evening snack. This eating pattern, too, will promote a deeper state of ketosis prior to the radiation.

My cancer experience did not include radiation, as there was no solid tumour present to receive the radiation "pulse." In my case, we were chasing individual cancer cells that might have escaped during the rupture and removal of the cancerous ovarian cyst. But if radiation is part of your recommended treatment plan, be assured that following a ketogenic diet can be just as powerful an intervention as it is during chemotherapy, maybe even more so. Remember those "cured" mice?

Alternative Therapies

There is a variety of cancer therapies currently in the "alternative health care" space that are not yet part of conventional medicine. It is not the role of this book to address these protocols, such as mistletoe therapy, hyperbaric oxygen therapy, and high-dose intravenous vitamin C therapy. These therapies are provided on a user-pay basis in many countries around the world, and hopefully rigorous scientific evidence will eventually be completed and published to allow them to be added to the arsenal of cancer-fighting treatments.

Within the world of conventional treatment, there is new work being done on immunotherapies, targeted genetic therapies, and PARP inhibitors (targeting enzymatic repair processes). Again, these therapies are being subjected to rigorous testing to ensure their safety and how well they actually work.

As far as we know, there's no reason why eating healthy low-carb whole foods and healthy fats would be contraindicated in any of these therapies. Improving your basic underlying health by choosing to eat in a way that reduces inflammation and keeps blood glucose and circulating growth factors low can only be beneficial. There's no published evidence to support this statement but common sense would suggest that this is so.

Part 4
Life Goes On...

Once Cancer Is Behind You

Getting cancer is sort of like becoming a parent. You are a parent as soon as you become pregnant. From that point on, you are forever a parent, even once your children are grown, launched into their own lives, even if they have died. You are never again not identified as a parent.

Likewise, once you are a person with cancer, you are never again NOT a person with cancer. You may take on the moniker of "cancer survivor" as one of your many labels but it never goes away. It changes your sense of self-identity just as much as becoming a parent does. You can say, "I had cancer" but the reality is that there's always the chance of recurrence lurking in the background; the thought remains, hiding in the corners of your brain.

Planning a big vacation for the coming year? There's that niggling thought again: What if I get sick before I go? What if the cancer comes back? Looking forward to retirement? There's a slightly different colour to your vision of that future, tinted by the presence of cancer in your past.

But this book, and this chapter, are not about being pessimistic or hopeless. We are POWERFUL BEYOND MEASURE! We have the knowledge and tools to make an impact on our future path. While there are no guarantees, making lifestyle changes, particularly around what we put into and onto our bodies, can make a big difference in how we go forward into our future.

This chapter will look at mindset, diet/intake, and lifestyle factors that will minimize your chances of a recurrence by making your body resistant to the formation and growth of tumours. Like sprinkling cayenne pepper among the plants in your garden to discourage pests, you are going to make the internal environment of your body inhospitable to cancer cells. Those cells, without a comfortable place to set up shop, will be targeted and destroyed by your own system in a wonderful housecleaning process called autophagy. The word literally means "eating oneself" and it's an apt description of how the process works. It happens inside individual cells and can lead to cellular death. **Autophagy can be compared to housecleaning. Sorting and culling and tidying stuff that shouldn't be left lying around.**

This is different from "apoptosis," a process of programmed cell death. It's one of the "hallmarks" of cancer cells that they can avoid apoptosis, thus not self-destroying when their genetic material is damaged. This leads to uncontrolled growth—a tumour.

The immune system also has a role to play in finding, identifying, and removing cancer cells. The immune system is a whole group of cells and body functions that act as the body's defense army. Keeping your immune system robust and focussed is a big part of staying healthy. When the immune system is malfunctioning and identifies normal parts of your own body as "invaders," it will attack and destroy—this is called an autoimmune disorder. Examples of common autoimmune diseases are lupus, inflammatory bowel diseases, rheumatoid arthritis, multiple sclerosis, type 1 diabetes, and Hashimoto's thyroiditis. Likewise, when the immune system is suppressed or underactive (such as when chemotherapy drugs damage bone marrow production) the body is left without defenses and is more susceptible to infections. Through optimal nutrition and lifestyle interventions, you can make a significant impact on the health of your immune system.

There's nothing like a health crisis to make a person focus on making beneficial changes in their behaviours. Although I had been eating low-carb and healthy fat (LCHF) for years before getting a cancer diagnosis, it was a whole new world once I started chemo. Being 100 percent compliant with a strict (<20g/day carb) ketogenic diet was easy when in that mindset. I said no to desserts that would otherwise have tempted me, no to every alcoholic beverage, no to potato chips and other salty treats, even no to sushi! Once chemo was over, however, I looked ahead and decided that there was a place in my world now for a bit more leniency and less "deprivation." I use that word carefully, as I don't find a keto diet particularly onerous.

Using high-fat, richly flavoured, umami-deep foods meets my needs for the most part and leaves me satisfied. But with summer just around the corner, I decided that I would once again allow a modest amount of sweet-tasting foods, possibly the occasional lower-carb alcoholic beverage and some starchier vegetables, such as sweet potatoes. Plus, summer fruits—I love peaches!

There is a balance to be found when choosing which behaviours to allow and not allow. That balance is between safety and joy. Safety meaning that you are not putting yourself at high risk of a bad outcome with your choice, such as smoking or eating commercially deep-fried foods. Joy meaning that you feel a heightened sense of happiness with life when you include certain things, such as eating a culturally important food—in my case, dressing/stuffing at Christmas, or a food you love, like sushi meals out with my husband.

So each person needs to find the place of balance that allows for them to have a joyful life but also to live without fear of recurrence being brought on by their behaviours. Where exactly that balance lies must be individually determined. Life, with or without cancer, is too short to be second-guessing every bite that goes into your mouth. Save your emotional and physical (and spiritual) energy for the parts of life that bring you joy.

Suggested post-chemo lifestyle choices to minimize the chances of recurrence:

- Continue to eat a moderate low-carb healthy fats (LCHF) diet. You can liberalize your carb intake so that you are not always in deep ketosis (>0.5 on the blood test meter) but rather that you dance around the edges of ketosis (0.2–0.5). For some, that might be about 50 g carb/day, for others up to 100 g carb/day. Don't worry about eating to your macros; simply eat adequately from your usual good food choices and make a conscious decision whether it's worth it to deviate from them when an opportunity comes along.
- Continue to emphasize the *quality* of your diet. At its most basic, avoid large quantities of added sugars and any quantity of industrial seed oils. This would translate into the following:
  - ¤ Only have a sweet item if it truly makes your heart sing...
  - ¤ Simply say NO to deep-fried fast foods or snack foods that

have come from a factory or fast food restaurant.

◻ Add real flavour to your meals with healthy fats, such as butter, olive oil, or avocados.

• Get adequate sleep. Sleep is emerging as one of the most important health determinants for physical health, mental health, prevention of illness and overall quality of life. It's something that we,
as a society, have ignored and even denigrated. It's become a point
of pride that one can "survive" on fewer hours of sleep or pull
an "all-nighter." In evolutionary terms, we are diurnal creatures,
designed to be awake and active in the light and sleep during the
dark periods. Modern life makes that hard. Do whatever is necessary to improve on your sleep patterns.

• Get outside. Real fresh air, real sunshine, and real contact with the
earth are all powerful stimulants of our feel-good hormones and
our immune systems. A practice known as forest-bathing is popular in Japan and is also being recognized in the rest of the world.
It has been studied for its ability to reduce stress hormone production, improve feelings of happiness, and free up creativity, as well
as lower heart rate and blood pressure, boost the immune system,
and accelerate recovery from illness. Until the last few hundred
years, even saying something like "get outside" would have been
ridiculous since most of life was lived outside, but in our modern
times, we have become dramatically disconnected from nature.

• Clean up your life to reduce exposure to nonnatural chemicals.
This has many parts, both environmental and in terms of what we
put into and onto our bodies. In our homes, that means getting
rid of air fresheners and strongly scented cleaners. Those scents are
all foreign chemicals that you're breathing into your body. Reduce
your myriad shower or bath products to one simple shampoo and
a bar of soap, maybe a conditioner if you have hair that needs it.
Choose as natural and low-scent of a product as you can find that
will still do the job. Go easy on the heavily scented laundry deter-
gents and dryer sheets—they just mean more chemicals entering
your body via your breath and your skin.

• Choose only organic products if you're going to reintroduce any
significant amount of grains into your diet. Doing so will remove

the contamination of your food products by glyphosate and other herbicides and pesticides. The whole GMO movement is mostly about making plants that can literally be bathed in these chemicals without them dying—not what you want in your body. Use organic bread, organic pasta, organic flour for baking, organic oatmeal, organic prepared breakfast cereals, and organic rice. Most of these foods have little or no place in an LCHF diet, but if you're buying them for occasional use or for regular use by other family members, make sure they are organic. Nowadays, this is not so hard to find and only minimally more expensive than regular grain products. Most supermarket chains have their own store brands (e.g. PC Organics, Our Compliments Organics).

- Continue to use fasting as a great cellular cleanup mechanism. Shorter fasts such as a 24-hour fast (from supper one night to supper the next night) or a 36-hour fast (from supper one night to breakfast the day after next), can be powerful promoters of cellular cleanup processes, such as autophagy and apoptosis. They can be done frequently, even several times weekly. You can establish a practice of fasting until suppertime every Monday and Friday, for example.

- Occasionally, do a longer fast—up to 72 hours, like you did during chemotherapy. A study published in 2014 showed that a three-day fast can essentially reset the immune system, providing many potential benefits (27). In his study, Dr. Valter Longo and colleagues at the University of Southern California found that fasting lowered white blood cell counts, which in turn triggered the immune system to start producing new white blood cells. Essentially a reboot to the entire system—fresh new cells. It won't be quite as easy as it was during chemo because you don't have the appetite-suppressing effects of feeling unwell, but use your bone broth as meal replacements and remember that hunger comes in waves and will pass. Stay busy and enjoy the fact that you have freed up several hours of time in each day that would otherwise be used for preparing, eating, and cleaning up from meals.

- Reintroduce your precancer activities and responsibilities—but don't just throw yourself back into everything that took up your time and energy before. Mindfully decide which activities would genuinely bring you satisfaction or joy, which you'd willingly take on as responsibilities, and which you now recognize as time- or energy-suckers and can simply refuse to resume. Cancer is the great cobweb clearer. Living a negatively stressful life has real and serious consequences for both physical and mental health. We were never meant to be chronically bathed in stress hormones. It's not a natural state that we have evolved to handle, and it affects both brain and body in bad ways. Find the balance of necessary work, joy-inducing activities, and peaceful downtime that resonates best with you.

- Resume physical activity but listen carefully to your body. Do not over-train or run your body down. After finishing chemo in May, I was determined that I would start running again and do a race of some sort by September of my chemo year. That was totally unrealistic and never happened. I walked, gardened, and rode my bike but never achieved running. Chemical residues and damage from the chemo will affect your body for months afterwards—don't expect instant results. Physical exercise is a form of stress on the body—that's how it works to improve our health—by stressing us (lungs, muscles, heart, etc.) so that we rebuild stronger for the next time. But asking for this adaptive rebuild in the post-chemo period is not good. Our rebuilding energy is still going into building us back up after the cancer experience. Overtraining can also have the effect of depressing your immune system function. That's why some marathon runners get sick right after their big race. Don't do it—you need your immune system functioning well to help reduce the chance of cancer recurrence.

- Keep a positive mindset. Stay emotionally and spiritually connected to your community, to your life and your activities. Practice prayer, positive intentions, attraction principles—whatever your particular choice may be for connecting to the larger energy of the Universe. Look for the silver linings in everything that happens. Give voice to your wishes, both out loud and in your head, then live your life in a way that will make those wishes manifest.

There *is* life after cancer, even though it's not life with no cancer in it. As with going through chemotherapy or other treatments, you are the master of your own fate in many ways and you can choose how you will respond to any situation. If things get tough, it's okay to sit down in the middle of the path and bawl your eyes out. But then, dry your eyes, get back on your feet, take a good look around at your situation, and start putting one foot in front of the other again.

I've had the following quote on my fridge for decades and it still resonates so strongly with me:

"The longer I live, the more I realize the impact of attitude on life. Attitude, to me, is more important than facts. It is more important than the past, the education, the money, than circumstances, than failure, than successes, than what other people think or say or do. It is more important than appearance, giftedness, or skill. It will make or break a company…a church…a home. The remarkable thing is we have a choice every day regarding the attitude we will embrace for that day. We cannot change our past…we cannot change the fact that people will act in a certain way. We cannot change the inevitable. The only thing we can do is play on the one string we have, and that is our attitude. I am convinced that life is 10% what happens to me and 90% of how I react to it. And so it is with you…we are in charge of our Attitudes."

— **Charles R. Swindoll**

Cancer As a Chronic Disease

Even *having* a discussion about cancer as a "chronic disease" and not a "terminal disease" shows how far cancer care has come in the past few decades. When cancer is assumed to be a battle to the death, the "War on Cancer," there can only be two outcomes: Winner or loser. Total remission or failure. Cure or death. It's a grim proposition…

However, there's a third path and that is the possibility of living with cancer for an extended period. Many people don't even know that this path exists. But current treatment options are now achieving success in putting cancer into either remission or at least a stable, non-advancing state and more "cancer patients" are becoming "cancer survivors."

My cancer, ovarian cancer, is one commonly held up as an example of a "chronic cancer" because of its high recurrence rate and also because those recurrences can often be managed so that the cancer journeyer is able to continue with life for a long time. Other examples of common chronic cancers are leukemia, lymphoma, prostate, and breast cancer.

As with other chronic diseases, such as multiple sclerosis or type 1 diabetes, the goal of extended treatment for cancer is to help patients live as well as possible for as long as possible. This involves ongoing treatment that's not meant to cure but to control progression and lead to disease "stability." Extended treatment options may include chemotherapy, immunotherapy, targeted therapy, radiation therapy, or hormone therapy.

In some circumstances, a cancer cannot be put into remission with the initial treatment plan of surgery, radiation, or chemotherapy. Even if remission is achieved, a cancer can recur, requiring further treatment. The idea of cancer as a chronic disease as opposed to a terminal one means that treatment options and lifestyle interventions are long-term changes.

If controlling a cancer's growth—making it into a stable, non-progressing health condition—is the goal, then it's obvious that dietary choices that continue to support the health of your overall body and that stress the cancer cells and make for inhospitable conditions are the best dietary choices to make. That brings us back to the LCHF, or ketogenic diet. On an ongoing basis, depriving your cancer cells of blood glucose spikes and fluctuations will make them less prone to growth. In addition, keeping your circulating insulin levels low will not feed their need for growth factors. If you can slow or stabilize cancer growth by these dietary and lifestyle interventions, you may require fewer of the other harsher treatments.

Like the diabetic who can reduce medications and insulin by restricting their carbohydrates, it might be possible to reduce the need for cancer-growth-limiting drugs or treatments if carb restriction can be maintained. Like a type 1 or type 2 diabetic, this is not a quick fix but rather a lifelong "new normal." The possible reduction in medication side effects and reduced costs would be worth it, though.

People with celiac disease will tell you that "cheating" on their gluten-free diet is totally not worth it—the consequences are both immediate (abdominal pain, raging diarrhea) and long term (intestinal gut lining damage and increased risk of bowel cancer in the future). Likewise, "cheating" regularly on a cancer-stabilizing LCHF or keto diet is not worth it, although you might not have the immediate negative feedback of the noncompliant celiac. Long term, you are feeding the cancer and making it harder for your treatment protocol to successfully stop growth.

Living with chronic cancer often requires long-term adherence to a medication regimen with nutritional side effects. Steroids, such as prednisone or dexamethasone, can cause elevated blood sugars, weight gain, increased appetite, poor skin integrity (you bruise or tear your skin more easily), and even type 2 diabetes severe enough to require treatment. Other drugs can cause ongoing constipation or diarrhea, gastric pain or reflux (heartburn), dry mouth, or numb and tingly extremities, including the tongue. All these factors can make sticking to a healthy diet more challenging.

Having chronic cancer can make you feel angry, scared, anxious, or sad. Doing something for yourself that gives you a feeling of control and empowerment over the situation is another reason to stick with your good dietary choices. Finding a support group, a counsellor, or a cancer survivor "buddy" will also help you to navigate this unknown future.

The idea of cancer as a chronic, manageable illness instead of a terminal win-or-lose disease is unknown to many people and so you might have to explain your situation to family, friends, and your support group. Your support circle, that gathered so valiantly around you in the initial push to "beat" your cancer, might drift away when the treatment turns into a years-long process instead of a few months of chemo or radiation. But keep in mind the type 1 diabetic or the celiac with a lifelong dietary intolerance. You have joined the ranks of the masses with a chronic illness. Management is the goal, living life to the fullest is the plan, and both are completely possible.

Part 5
Easy Keto Recipes —
Basics and Good Substitutes

Bone Broth

Focaccia-Style Low-Carb Bread

Magic Keto Flax/Psyllium Bread – for Constipation Relief

KFC-Style Breading

Fathead Pizza

Keto Egg Roll in a Bowl

Creamy Keto Mushroom Soup

Instant Pot Spaghetti Squash Casserole

Cauliflower Mac 'n' Cheese with Bacon

Roasted Lower-Carb Vegetables

Chicken Liver Pâté

Sesame Seed Crispy Crackers

Keto Crack-ola

Healthy Oil Mayonnaise

Fat Bombs

Chia Seed Fruit Jam

Mason Jar Ice Cream

Bone Broth – The Fasting Meal Replacer

There's nothing like a hot mug of bone broth to make you feel like you've had a meal while fasting. If lunch time or supper time rolls around and your body is telling you that you are expected to eat something, bone broth will be your best friend. In fact, it is meal-ish enough that you can sit down with others and have your broth with minimal comment.

Late in the day, coffee may be a bad idea. Even decaf can have a stimulating effect, bothering your sleep. Same for black and green teas. The caffeine in both can be enough to make settling at night difficult. That's where bone broth works so well. It's hot, sending the signal that it's a meal, not a snack. It's savoury, another satiety trigger that says "meal," not "treat." And it's salty and full of minerals that your body needs in exaggerated amounts during a fast or while in ketosis. Most of the symptoms of "keto flu" can be relieved by adding adequate fluids and minerals.

Bone broth was key to enabling me to fast during chemo treatments. The first day of each fast, a Wednesday, was always a workday, and I have a well-entrenched pattern of meals and snacking at work. In addition, I eat lunch around a table with coworkers and not attending isn't really an option. So I would take my glass container of bone broth to work, warm it in the microwave until it was piping hot, and eat most of it with a spoon. That took most of the lunch hour and had me behaving just like everyone else. Of course, they all knew that I was fasting for the treatment the next day, but it wasn't as weird as sitting there just watching the others and not as isolating as avoiding the lunchroom altogether.

The second serving would travel to London with me. I would sip herbal tea from my thermos during the three-hour drive down—I always drove the whole way myself because I wouldn't be up to sharing the driving duties the next day. We'd stop for shawarma on the way through the city and I'd watch my hubby enjoy his meal while sipping my tea. When we got to the hotel (usually between 8:00 and 9:00 p.m.), I'd warm up my jar of bone broth and have my "supper."

The day of chemo didn't seem to require bone broth, probably because I kind of lost my appetite once things were underway. The drive home after chemo was usually accompanied by herbal tea, and the following day, I didn't have much appetite either. By afternoon, I'd be rallying and planning my post-meal dinner at the end of the 72 hours. Bone broth went onto the back burner until the next time.

Bone broth is dead easy to make but some companies are jumping on the bandwagon of providing it as a premade product. I will not make specific brand recommendations in this book, as they will quickly become outdated, but a search of the internet or a question posed in a keto/low-carb/fasting group will quickly yield recommendations for brands, flavours, and availability. Instead, I am going to try and convince you of how simple it is to make your own and hence know the quality of what you're getting. Packaged chicken or beef "broth" is not an adequate substitution. It's a manufactured "food-like substance," as Michael Pollen would call it, and is full of chemical crap.

It's so much cheaper to make your own as well. Although bone broth is becoming a "thing," bones are still dirt cheap if you know where to look. If you patronize a butcher shop or farm store of any type, you can talk to the staff about getting cast-off bones, such as chicken backs, the part left after the breasts and leg quarters have been cut off. You can buy great bones at a good grocery store but you will pay a premium price for them, as bones are becoming much more popular.

Another great alternative is to have a large Ziploc bag always on the go in your freezer. Each time you eat a meal with bones left over (chicken, pork chops, beef ribs, or lamb shank), scrape the leftover bone and gristle and fatty bits into the bag. Try and avoid adding lots of barbeque sauce or other flavours—this may involve rinsing the bones before adding them to the bag. When it's time to make bone broth, you will have a collection of precooked bones to enrich your pot.

If your goal is collagen-rich broth, you should focus on adding some "joints" and skin, both rich in connective tissue. Think shank bones, pork hocks, chicken feet, and the white gristle at the ends of the chicken bones. The grotty bits that are not a usual part of our North American diet but are commonly used in other parts of the world.

If starting with raw bones, be sure and roast them first to add some browning to the tissues and greatly enhance the flavour and colour of the finished broth. Bones can simply be spread out on a roasting pan or baking sheet that has sides and placed in the oven for up to an hour—depending on the bones—until they are looking and smelling roasted. Because there's little actual meat tissue, this doesn't take as long as cooking a piece of meat. I have often taken chicken backs straight out of the freezer, placed them in the oven at 375 F on a roasting pan for 20 minutes or so, then removed the pan and separated the chicken carcasses into separate pieces (impossible to do easily while they are frozen). Then I'd put them back into the oven for another 20 minutes until they're well roasted and crispy-skinned.

Once well cooked, place the bones along with all the meat juices and rendered fat from the baking pan into the broth pot—either a large stock pot on the stovetop, a slow cooker, or an Instant Pot. You can also add the contents of your precooked bones bag, right from the freezer and maybe also include an onion, a stalk of celery, and a carrot for flavour. Also, add a splash (a couple of tablespoons) of apple cider vinegar to the pot. Don't worry—you will not end up with acidic broth. It's thought that the small amount of acidity helps to soften and extract additional minerals from the bones as the broth cooks. Wait until the broth is done to add salt and pepper.

That's about it…. If using a pot on the stove, bring to a boil, turn down to your lowest simmer, put on the lid, and check the fluid level before you go to bed, top up if it makes you feel better, then sleep the night away and wake up to the rich smell of broth cooking.

A slow cooker will also take 18–24 hours to produce a rich bone broth. Watch it to ensure that it doesn't need to be topped up with water before bed.

Alternatively, you can cook bone broth in an Instant Pot. Add the vegetables and bones to the inner steel liner of the Instant Pot, then fill up to the MAX line with cold water. Don't use hot water from your tap—it's been through who-knows-what in the hot water tank. Add your splash of apple cider vinegar and then close the lid, set the vent to seal, and push the Soup/Broth button. Adjust timing to two hours. And walk away…

It will take a while for the Instant Pot to heat up with so much cold water, so don't worry about it. And it will also take quite a while for the pot to finally cool enough after the cooking time for a natural release. Again, walk away…easiest thing ever.

Finishing your broth involves picking out the biggest of the bones with tongs or a slotted spoon to make it safer to strain so much hot liquid. Once you have the big chunks removed, pour your hot broth (very carefully, please!) through a strainer into a large pot or bowl for chilling. I use a pasta colander—it doesn't have to be a super fine metal mesh strainer. Work in your sink so that you don't have to lift the heavy pots higher than necessary—there's a definite risk of splashing or scalding with this process. Add some salt and pepper at this point—season to taste.

Put the entire bowl or pot of the strained broth into the fridge to chill for several hours or overnight. Once fully cold, a fat layer will form on the surface of the broth. This might be mushy soft in the case of poultry broth or quite solid in the case of meat broth. Remove as much fat as you can (you can discard it—all the good stuff is in the broth) and then pour your (hopefully) jiggly bone broth into containers for storage. Glass mason jars are great for refrigerator storage of broth that you are likely to use in the coming week but glass will crack in the freezer, thus wasting your precious broth and potentially causing quite a mess. For freezer storage, I have found that 750 ml/3 cup plastic storage containers are excellent. Because I am pouring a cold fluid into them, I have no concerns about plastic chemical leakage into my broth. Obviously, do not warm your broth in these containers—always switch to glass or ceramic or a pot for heating. Plastic containers can leach chemicals into the contents when microwaved or when in contact with hot food.

A 750 ml/3 cup container of bone broth is just about the right size to get through one 72-hour chemo fast. I would have two 250 ml/1 cup servings on Day 1 of my fast, as "lunch" and "supper," then use the last cup on Day 3 of the fast, to help me get through to my post-fast meal at suppertime.

The 3-cup serving size is also great for using as a base for homemade soups. Check out my Creamy Keto Mushroom Soup recipe for a favourite comfort food.

Focaccia-Style Low-Carb Bread

Makes 12–15 slices. Can be cut into larger or smaller pieces depending on the purpose.

INGREDIENTS

- 2 cups seed or nut meal (such as flax meal, ground chia seeds, or almond meal or any combination of these that makes 2 cups) *don't use high-carb, wheat-free flours
- 1 tbsp baking powder
- 1 tsp salt
- 2–3 envelopes of Stevia or other accepted sweetener (more can be added if making sweet-style bread)
- 5 eggs, beaten
- ½ cup water
- ⅓ cup extra light olive oil, avocado oil, or melted coconut oil

Preheat oven to 350 F. Prepare a pan (a 10x15-inch pan with sides works best) with oiled parchment paper or a silicone mat.

In a large bowl, whisk seed/nut meal, baking powder, salt, and sweetener.

Whisk together the eggs, water, and oil, then add to the dry ingredients and combine well. Make sure to break up any obvious strings of egg white.

Let batter set for 2–3 minutes to thicken up some. (Leaving it longer makes it difficult to spread.)

Pour batter onto the prepared pan. Spread it away from the centre and level it into a rectangle 1 or 2 inches away from the sides of the pan (you can go all the way to the edge but it will be thinner).

Bake for about 20 minutes, until it springs back when you touch the top and/or is visibly browning.

Let cool and then cut into whatever size slices you want. A pizza cutter works great—it's quite soft.

VARIATIONS

You can add either savoury spices (such as Italian spice mix, garlic, or onion powder) or sweet spices (cinnamon, ginger, cloves) to the dry ingredients. You can also sprinkle sesame or poppy seeds on the top before baking. Everything-but-the-bagel seasoning mix is also nice sprinkled on top. A handful of chopped pecans in the batter adds nice texture. The sliced bread freezes very well.

NUTRITION INFORMATION

Portion: two slices

Approximately 300 kcals, 1 g net carbs, 10.7 g fibre, 11 g protein and 23 g fat. Over 75 percent calories from fat. This analysis is based on half almond flour and half ground chia seeds. Different nutmeal and seed mixtures will result in slightly different values.

Magic Keto Flax/Psyllium Bread – for Constipation Relief

This is a modification of the low-carb, focaccia-style bread that I have been making for several years, usually using other low-carb seed and nut meals, such as almond meal, pecan meal, or ground chia seeds. But when the rubber hits the road, flax and psyllium are the best sources of both soluble and insoluble fibres for bulking stools and attracting and holding onto water in the large bowel.

Ingredients
- 1¾ cups flax meal
- ½ cup psyllium husk
- 1 tbsp baking powder
- 1 tsp salt
- 2–3 envelopes of Stevia or other noncaloric natural sweetener
- 5 eggs, beaten
- ½ cup water
- ⅓ cup of extra light olive oil, avocado oil, or melted coconut oil

Preparation
Preheat oven to 350 F. Prepare a pan. A 10×15" baking pan works best. Line with oiled parchment paper or a silicon mat. In a large bowl, mix all dry ingredients with a whisk to remove any lumps. In another bowl, add eggs, oil, and water and whisk thoroughly to eliminate any obvious strings of egg white. Add egg mixture to dry ingredients and stir well. Let batter

sit for 2–3 minutes to thicken up but not too long or it becomes hard to spread. Pour batter onto prepared pan and use a wet spatula to flatten out the mound until it's about ⅓" thick and level, then shape into a rectangle for best browning and easy portioning.

Bake for 20 minutes, or until it springs back when you touch the top, and/or is visibly browning. Let cool and the cut into about 15–18 slices. A pizza cutter works great. Store in the fridge and use two slices daily for bowel management. Freezes very well.

NUTRITIONAL INFORMATION:
    Portion: two slices
    245 kcals, 0.3 g net carbs, 9 g fibre, 7 g protein, and 20 g fat. About 80 percent calories from fat.

KFC-Style Breading

Use this breading mix on chicken wings, drumsticks, thighs, or strips of breast meat to make "chicken fingers."

- 1 cup almond meal/flour
- ½ tsp ginger
- ½ tsp parsley
- 1 tsp paprika
- ¼ tsp chili powder
- ½ tsp sage
- ½ tsp dry mustard powder
- ¼ tsp Chinese Five Spice (this is a blend of the traditionally sweet spices cinnamon and cloves, plus fennel seeds, anise, and peppercorns—adds interesting complexity but can be omitted if you don't have it)
- ½ tsp basil
- Salt and pepper to taste

Preheat oven to 350 F.

Mix all ingredients together in a large zipper-style freezer bag. Drop in chicken pieces, seal bag, and roll around until all of the chicken skin has been coated by the spice mix.

In a large casserole or baking pan, pour olive or avocado oil until bottom of dish is generously covered. Place the chicken pieces in the olive oil, turning them so the breaded surfaces are covered.

Bake in oven for 45 minutes. Turn the chicken pieces a couple of times to crisp up all sides.

If you are taking all those spices off the shelf anyways, why not make lots? This recipe can be easily doubled or tripled and stored for ready use. Keep a large batch ready in a jar, then just throw a half cup or so into a bag for a quick worknight supper. Keep your stash safely away from raw poultry—only take what you will need for that meal. This is a great time and money saver if you are only cooking small quantities of chicken at a time.

This recipe will add a negligible amount of carbohydrates to the chicken, and nutrition information will vary depending on the chicken pieces used and amount of oil.

Fathead Pizza

I can't take any credit for this recipe. It's all over the internet but comes originally from the website Ditch the Carbs (ditchthecarbs.com). It's a wonderful solid pizza crust, pick-up-able, tasty. You can't eat endlessly of this pizza as the high fat content of the crust makes it very filling. It's a simple, no rise, one bowl recipe that you can prepare while the oven is heating.

INGREDIENTS
- 1¾ cups grated or shredded mozzarella cheese (can be purchased or grated at home)
- ¾ cup almond flour
- 2 tbsp cream cheese
- 1 egg
- Pinch of salt to taste
- ½ tsp dried rosemary/Italian seasoning/garlic powder or other favourite herbs as desired (optional)

Preheat the oven to 425 F.

Mix shredded cheese and almond flour together in a microwavable bowl. Add cream cheese. Microwave on High for 1 minute.

Stir the semi-melted batter then microwave on High for another 30 seconds.

Add the egg, salt, and seasonings and mix gently.

Place a sheet of parchment paper on your counter large enough for the finished pizza. Dump the dough onto the sheet and cover with another sheet of parchment paper. Using your hands or a rolling pin, press the dough into a circular pizza shape. Work fairly quickly so that the mixture doesn't harden. If it does, just microwave again for 10–20 seconds (no lon-ger—you don't want to cook the egg).

Remove the top sheet of parchment paper and transfer the shell to a baking sheet, pizza pan, or pizza stone with the bottom sheet still under-neath.

Bake for 12–15 minutes, until browned. There will be oil bubbling in the shell—be careful when removing from the oven.

Remove from oven and add toppings. One pizza will hold about half of a small can of prepared pizza sauce (these will contain a small amount of sugar, plus the carbohydrates from the tomatoes, but the amount used is modest.) Add pepperoni or other precooked meats (ham, bacon, crumbled sausage, shredded chicken) and any low-carb vegetables that you like. Note that the second cooking time is not adequate to cook raw meat. Sprinkle with a light coating of additional cheese if desired (mozzarella, Parmesan, feta).

Return to oven and bake again for 5–8 minutes depending on your top-pings and how cooked you like them. Watch for overbrowning of exposed crust if you cook past 5 minutes.

Remove from oven and allow to sit for one minute just to cool off the very hot oils in the pizza and crust before cutting with a pizza roller or knife.

Enjoy!

Nutrition Information (for the crust alone)

Portion: a quarter of the pizza

305 kcals, 25 g fat, 6 g carbs, 16.5 g protein. About 74 percent calories from fat.

Keto Egg Roll in a Bowl

This Asian-inspired cabbage mix is designed to resemble the insides of an eggroll. Delicious without the deep fried (in horrible fats) carb-containing shell.

INGREDIENTS

- 1 lb ground pork (not sausage, fresh, unseasoned pork). You can easily use ground beef instead, as it's much easier to find.
- ½–1 head (about 8–10 cups) cabbage, thinly sliced into long strands (depending on size and density of cabbage). Easy to do with a mandoline or slicing blade on a food processor.
- 1 onion, thinly sliced into rings or slivers
- 1 tbsp (or more to taste) roasted sesame oil
- ¼ cup soy sauce, tamari, or liquid aminos
- 1 clove garlic, minced
- 1 tsp ground ginger
- 1 tbsp fresh ginger, minced (optional, but nice)
- 2 tbsp chicken broth
- 2 stalks of green onion, chopped
- Salt and pepper to taste

Brown ground meat in a very large pan or wok over a medium heat.

Add sesame oil and onion to pan, stir to combine, and continue to cook until onion softens.

Mix soy sauce, garlic, chicken broth, and ground ginger together in a small bowl. Add the fresh ginger if using.

Add the cabbage to the wok, then pour over the contents of the seasonings bowl and stir to mix the sauce throughout and coat the vegetables evenly. Continue cooking over medium heat, stirring frequently, until cabbage is desired softness.

Season with salt and black pepper to taste. Additional sesame oil can be drizzled over the finished dish, if desired, to intensify the flavour. Garnish with chopped green onions to serve.

NUTRITIONAL INFORMATION:

Portion: a sixth of the recipe

235 kcals, 6 g net carbs, 3 g fibre, 16 g protein, and 15 g fat. About 60 percent calories from fat. This will vary depending on which meat you use and its fat content.

Creamy Keto Mushroom Soup

True comfort food…

INGREDIENTS

- ¼ cup butter
- 5–6 cups coarsely chopped mushrooms (white, brown, Portobello—your preference)
- 1 medium onion, finely chopped
- 1 clove garlic, minced
- ½ tsp salt
- ½ tsp black pepper
- ¼–½ tsp dried thyme
- 3 cups bone broth (or a 3–4 cup carton of commercial chicken broth)
- 1 cup coffee cream (10–18%)
- 1 cup heavy whipping cream (32%)
- 4 oz (half brick) cream cheese
- 2 tbsp of sherry, bourbon, whisky, or rum—a sweetish tasting but carb-free liquor

In a large, heavy-bottomed saucepan, melt butter, then add mushrooms, onion, and garlic. Cook gently until tender, about 10 minutes. Add salt, pepper, and thyme, cook for another minute. Add chicken broth and cream cheese (cut into chunks). Bring to a boil, stirring to break up the cream cheese. Reduce heat to a simmer and let cook for 20 minutes. Add the cream and the liquor and continue to simmer for another 20 minutes, stirring frequently.

This recipe will make about four generous meal-sized bowls of soup. Because of the high fat content, it's very satisfying, unlike commercial soups.

Note: You could swap out the coffee cream for milk if you are not overly concerned with the carb content, but be sure to use the heavy whipping cream for the satiety-producing fat content. It will change up the carb count with a few extra grams of lactose sugars but this is not a major concern. According to USDA and Canadian Nutrient Files:

- heavy whipping cream – 7 g carb/cup
- 18% coffee cream – 9 g/cup
- 10% half and half cream – 11 g/cup
- homogenised milk – 12 g/cup
- 2% milk – 12 g/cup

In other words, use what you have in the house…

Also note: Don't skip the liquor. It adds an amazing depth of flavour to the soup, contributes to the umami richness of the mushrooms, adds a touch of sweetness without added sugar, and takes the soup to the next level. The original recipe suggested sherry but I never have that in the house. I have used non-smoky whiskey, bourbon, or rum with great results. The alcohol burns off completely in the cooking process, leaving the flavour behind.

NUTRITIONAL INFORMATION:

Portion: a quarter of the recipe

315 kcals, 8 g net carbs, 10 g total carbs, 10 g protein, 26 g fat. About 74 percent calories from fat.

Instant Pot Spaghetti Squash Casserole

Makes 4–6 large servings, depending on size of squash
- 1 large spaghetti squash, 3–4 lbs
- ½ lb bacon, sliced into small pieces
- 2 cups fresh peas, pea pods, sliced green beans, fresh spinach, or any combination of these
- ½ tsp salt
- ¼ tsp black pepper
- 1 tsp oregano
- ½ tsp garlic powder
- 6–8 oz full-fat cream cheese
- ¾ cup Parmesan cheese

INSTANT POT INSTRUCTIONS

Pierce spaghetti squash with paring knife all over, then place whole into Instant Pot with 1 cup water. Close and seal lid and set for 11 minutes on Pressure Cook. Allow 10 minutes natural release then remove pressure valve and take squash out to cutting board. Carefully slice open, remove seeds, shred the squash fibres, and return to Instant Pot.

Meanwhile, fry the bacon until crisp. Save the bacon fat in the pan. Chop the block of cream cheese into smaller pieces.

Add all other ingredients, including the bacon fat, to Instant Pot, except the Parmesan cheese. Stir to start cream cheese melting into the hot water. Cook on slow cooker setting for 1 hour, add Parmesan, and cook for another 30 minutes.

Serve with additional Parmesan cheese for sprinkling, if desired.

Slow Cooker instructions

Pierce spaghetti squash with paring knife all over, then place whole into crockpot with 1 cup water. Cover and cook on high for 4 hours. Once soft, remove and cut open and scoop out seeds, then shred squash fibres and return to the hot water in the crock pot.

Meanwhile, fry the bacon until crisp. Save the bacon fat in the pan. Chop the block of cream cheese into smaller pieces.

Add all other ingredients, including the bacon fat, to the crock pot, except the Parmesan cheese. Stir to start cream cheese melting into the hot water. Cook on high for 1 hour, add Parmesan, and cook for another 30 minutes.

Serve with additional Parmesan for sprinkling, if desired.

Nutritional Information:

Portion: a sixth of the recipe

325 kcals, 17 g net carbs, 5 g fibre, 13 g protein, 21 g fat. About 60% calories from fat.

Cauliflower Mac 'n' Cheese with Bacon

A great substitute for the all-time comfort food, macaroni and cheese. Hits all the same buttons…

Ingredients

- 1 large head cauliflower
- 6 oz cream cheese, cut into ½-inch cubes (¾ of the large block)
- ¾ cup sour cream
- 1 tsp Dijon mustard
- ¼ cup minced green onions (optional, but nice)
- ¼ cup Parmesan cheese, grated
- 6 slices bacon (or more to taste)
- 1 cup grated sharp cheddar cheese

Instructions

Preheat oven to 350 F. Spray or grease a large glass casserole dish with olive oil or nonstick spray.

Wash and core the cauliflower, break the head into even-sized florets for cooking. Boil in salted water until tender but not mushy soft—poke with a fork after 5 minutes to check for tenderness.

Drain well and return to pot. Mash with potato masher, leaving it chunky.

While cauliflower is cooking, fry bacon until crisp and crumbly, slice green onions (if using), and cube the cream cheese. Reserve the bacon fat to add to the recipe.

Add cream cheese, sour cream, mustard, bacon, green onions, and Parmesan cheese to the cauliflower mash. Fold together gently to mix all ingredients, start the cream cheese melting, and keep the cauliflower chunks intact.

Spoon out the creamy cauliflower mix into the prepared baking dish, smooth the top, and sprinkle with the cheddar cheese. You can reserve a bit of the bacon to sprinkle on top as well if you wish. Cover and bake 20–25 minutes, until hot and bubbly, then uncover and bake an additional 10 minutes until cheese is slightly browned. Serve hot.

This recipe can also be chilled, then sliced into single portions for workday meals. It reheats beautifully in a glass container (never plastic!).

NUTRITIONAL INFORMATION:

Portion: a fifth of the recipe

250 kcals, 8 g net carbs, 3 g fibre, 12 g protein, 18 g fat. About 70 percent calories from fat.

Roasted Lower-Carb Vegetables

When I went lower carb, I wanted to continue roasting veggies to bring out their wonderful flavours and natural sweetness, but low-carb, high-water-content foods behave differently than starchy root vegetables. Well, I'm here to tell you that they can be just as delicious and beautiful on the plate. I'm talking about red/green/yellow/orange bell peppers, cauliflower, broccoli, asparagus, fennel, celery, mushrooms, green beans, Brussel sprouts, cabbage, or onions.

There are a few tricks to roasting low-carb veggies. First of all, the temperature in the oven must be significantly higher than for starchy winter root vegetables. While starchy veggies do best at 350 F, the low-carb veggies need a much higher temperature, usually doing best at 400–425 F. They also take significantly less time to cook, 30–45 minutes vs. 60–90 minutes for the starchy mixes. Both versions benefit from using parchment paper underneath them. (I still marvel that I made it into my mid-fifties before discovering the wonders of parchment paper!)

The beauty of cooking vegetables this way is that you can make up massive quantities at once and use a wide variety of different flavours and colours, boosting nutrient content while adding beauty to your plate. You can batch cook a week's worth of lunches this way as well.

INGREDIENTS
- 2 red peppers cut into chunks
- 1 head of cauliflower cut into large florets
- 1 fennel bulb, sliced
- brown mushrooms (stems removed)

- 1 lb asparagus
- ¼ cup olive oil
- ½ tsp salt
- ¼ tsp pepper
- ½ tsp garlic powder
- 1 heaped tbsp of dried green herbs, such as an Italian or Greek herb blend, or Herbes de Provence

INSTRUCTIONS

Preheat oven to 400 F.

Wash and cut up your vegetables into largish, bite-sized chunks. Place in large bowl and drizzle with olive oil to coat evenly. Sprinkle with salt, pepper, garlic powder, and your dried green herbs of choice.

Spread out on a parchment paper-lined baking sheet (preferably one with sides), as evenly and thinly as possible. Use multiple pans if necessary. Bake in oven, stirring gently after 20–30 minutes and tasting a piece or two for desired doneness. They will shrink down a bit with cooking. Remove from oven and, using the parchment paper as a funnel, pour the mixture into a serving bowl.

For added "sophistication," drizzle with balsamic vinegar.

Chicken Liver Pâté

If you're committed to eating nose-to-tail, as our ancestors did, getting liver into your diet is important. Organ meats are nutritional powerhouses and liver is the KING of organs. But many people have lived their whole lives without ever experiencing liver and many more are "grossed out" by the texture or intense flavour. This is unfortunate, as liver is the original superfood.

The same people who can't bear to even think about liver will, however, often love liver pâté. This is a great recipe with a rich buttery texture and umami flavour with a touch of sweetness thanks to the addition of the brandy.

INGREDIENTS

- 1 lb fresh chicken livers, cleaned
- 1 cup milk
- ½ cup cold unsalted butter, cut into pieces
- 1 cup chopped onion
- 2 tsp minced garlic
- 2 tbsp green peppercorns, drained
- 2 bay leaves
- 1 tsp chopped fresh thyme leaves
- ½ tsp salt
- ½ tsp freshly ground black pepper
- ¼ cup cognac or brandy

INSTRUCTIONS

In a bowl, soak the livers in milk for 2 hours. Drain well.

In a large skillet, melt ¼ cup of your butter over a medium heat. Add onions and cook until soft, about 3 minutes. Add the garlic and cook until fragrant. Add the chicken livers, 1 tablespoon of peppercorns, herbs, salt, and pepper. Cook, stirring until the livers are browned on the outside and still slightly pink on the inside, about 5 minutes. Add the cognac/brandy and cook until most of the liquid is evaporated and the livers are cooked through but still tender.

Remove from heat and let cool slightly. Remove the bay leaves and discard.

In a food processor, purée the liver mixture. Add the remaining butter in pieces and pulse to blend. Fold in the remaining 1 tablespoon of peppercorns and adjust seasonings to taste.

Pack the pâté into small ramekins or jars, about 4 oz each. Cover and refrigerate until firm, at least 6 hours. Use within a few days or freeze for future meals.

NUTRITIONAL INFORMATION:

For a sixth recipe: 295 kcals, 3 g net carbs, 19 g protein, 20 g fat. About 70 percent calories from fat. Fabulous source of bioavailable iron at 9 grams per serving.

Sesame Seed Crispy Crackers

This is the ultimate keto answer to the need for crispy crunch. As a lifelong cracker eater, this recipe has been a godsend. One batch makes lots of crackers that store well in an airtight container at room temperature. Like most low-carb, grain-type foods, these are much denser and more filling than regular crackers. Four to five is a satisfying serving.

My ultimate comfort food snack is crackers and cheese, preferably old cheddar. These crackers fit the bill beautifully. I have been known to have crackers and cheese for breakfast, lunch, or snack. Or alongside a bowl of soup for supper. There's just no bad time for crackers and cheese...

The secret to the wonderful crunch is the triple baking process. It allows the crackers to properly dry out. Believe me, it's worth the wait. Whip them up after supper, turn off the oven before you go to bed, and wake up to perfect crackers in the morning!

The other big bonus with this recipe is that it doesn't include nut products. That makes it much more affordable than many keto baking items.

INGREDIENTS

- 1½ cups sesame seeds (raw)
- 1 tbsp psyllium husk (important for texture—don't skip this ingredient)
- ¼ cup pumpkin seeds
- ½ cup sunflower seeds
- 1 cup grated Parmesan cheese (can be substituted with up to ½ cup Asiago or other grated strongly flavoured dry-hard cheese)
- 1 tbsp Everything but the Bagel Seasoning (or substitute with 1

tsp garlic powder, 1 tsp dried minced onion or onion powder, ½
tsp large crystal salt, 1 tsp poppy seeds if desired)
- 2 large eggs
- ½ cup cold water

INSTRUCTIONS

Preheat oven to 350 F. Prepare a large baking sheet by lining it with
parchment paper.

Mix all dry ingredients in a large bowl.

Add eggs and water, mix to combine.

Pour the batter onto the prepared baking sheet. With wet hands or a
wet spatula, pat the batter down until it's a large rectangle about ¼ inch
thick.

Bake for 25 minutes. The top should be golden brown.

Remove from the oven and turn temperature down to 200 F. Cut the
cracker sheet into small rectangles. A pizza cutter wheel works great for
this. Make your crackers 1½ inches or so on a side. My pan usually yields
about 42–48 crackers (cut 6 x 7). If you are able, wiggle each cracker slightly to give airspace between them. This allows for better crisping in the
second baking.

Return to the oven and bake for an additional 2 hours.

When done, turn off the heat and leave the pan in the oven overnight
(this is the third "bake"). This allows for a very slow cooling and release of
any remaining moisture.

Next morning, the crackers can be enjoyed or stored in an airtight container at room temperature. If they are stored when even the slightest bit
warm, they will soften.

The original recipe, from which this was adapted, indicated that they
could be stored in the freezer for up to three months. Yeah, right! Not in
my world…

NUTRITIONAL INFORMATION:

(Per cracker) 45 kcals, 1 g net carbs, 2 g protein, and 4 g fat.

Keto Crack-ola

There are certain things that make sticking to a ketogenic diet easier. As much as I love meat, eggs, healthy fats, and vegetables, there are times when I can't face another egg and I just want something that at least resembles a grain product, like bread, cookies, or cereal. And sometimes, you just need something a bit sweet. Or something crunchy.

That's where this granola comes in. It's sweet, thanks to non-nutritive natural sweeteners. It's crunchy, thanks to the long baking time. It can be eaten dry, like a cookie substitute. It can be a cereal, swamped in almond milk, cream, yogurt, or kefir.

The basis of the cereal is nuts and seeds. High in healthy fats, low in carbs, gluten free, paleo, vegetarian (not vegan)—it hits all the right notes. It's also freakishly delicious and very easy to overeat. Ask me how I know…

I decided that since it's granola-like, but not grain-based, it needed a new name. Others have called it No-la, since it's no-grain-ola, and I thought of Nut-ola, but do you know what it really is? It's freaking crack—that's what it is! The first time I made a batch (and a batch is big!), I ate the entire thing in a few days. Breakfast with almond milk, afternoon snack as sweet, crunchy finger food, evening snack with almond milk again, or possibly dry with tea. Just way too much. So it became known in my mind as Crack-ola. And that has stuck.

My first batch was loosely based on the following recipe but was made using the ingredients I happened to have in my cupboards that day. When making it a second time, I endeavoured to measure and write down what

I was doing. It was a bit different than the first time but just as good. So you can make it exactly as in the recipe below, or just use what you have, or your favourite mix of nuts and seeds, but keep the glaze and the cooking method the same.

Here's the original recipe from Gnom-Gnom Paleo. Thanks to Paola for sharing her recipe and cooking method: https://www.gnom-gnom.com/top-secret-grain-free-keto-granola/.

And here's mine…

INGREDIENTS

- 1 cup almonds, whole, slivered, sliced, or a combo
- 1 cup pecan pieces
- ½ cup sunflower seeds
- ½ cup pumpkin seeds
- ½ cup coconut flakes, unsweetened
- ½ cup chia seeds
- ½ cup hemp hearts, raw
- 6 tbsp sesame seeds
- 8 tbsp non-nutritive natural sweetener of choice (Stevia, erythritol, monk fruit, or some combination)
- 1 tbsp molasses or maple syrup
- 1 tsp cinnamon
- 2 egg whites
- Sea salt for sprinkling

INSTRUCTIONS

Preheat oven to 250 F. Prepare a large baking sheet with sides by lining it with parchment paper.

In a dry frying pan, toast the almonds, watching very closely to prevent burning. They will develop a rich smell. In a large bowl combine toasted almonds, pecans, sunflower seeds, pumpkin seeds, chia seeds, and hemp hearts and mix together.

In the same dry frying pan, toast the sesame seeds until richly fragrant, stirring frequently and watching closely to prevent burning. Add to a food processor or blender with sweetener, molasses or maple syrup, and cinnamon. Blend, scraping down sides frequently, to pulverize the sesame seeds. Add sweet mix to the seed bowl and mix well.

Beat the two egg whites with an electric mixer until soft peaks form. Fold into the nut and seed mix and stir until all the ingredients are glazed with the egg white. This will adhere the sweet mix to the nuts and seeds. It should all look vaguely damp. Sprinkle with sea salt.

Spread the granola mix out evenly on the prepared pan and bake in the oven for 1 hour. Allow to cool completely, then break into pieces and store in a Ziploc bag or other airtight container to keep it crunchy.

NUTRITIONAL INFORMATION:

Portion: about a third to a half of a cup, depending on which nuts/seeds you added.

270 kcals, 5 g net carbs, 7 g fibre, 8 g protein, and 23 g fat. Over 75 percent calories from fat.

A word about sweeteners. I used a golden monk fruit sweetener from Lakanto but any preferred sweetener that measures like sugar will work. A brown sugar-style substitute gives the richest "caramelized" effect. And the small amount of real sweetener, whether it's molasses or maple syrup, adds a delicious depth of flavour and some extra stickiness to the mix. Don't skip it—it's worth the few extra carbs per serving.

Healthy Oil Mayonnaise

I love mayonnaise and it's one of the very few sources of industrial seed oils that I still allow in my diet or my household. I have found avocado oil mayonnaise at the local health food store, for the steep price of $14.99. I didn't like it at all—it has a very flat flavour. Disappointed, I went back to my beloved Hellmann's Real Mayonnaise, with olive oil, feeling somewhat virtuous (for the olive oil part) and somewhat guilty (about the canola oil part). It's a blend with canola oil—I know that—but I wasn't aware of the actual ratio of that blend until I had a client who was a very inquisitive sort and she called the company and asked. The olive oil comprises a measly 8% of the oil content of the "Olive Oil Mayo." The other 92% is canola oil—highly processed, deodorized, and a genetically modified (GM) crop. This makes sense given the relative costs of the two oils.

Canola is a major North American oilseed crop. Approximately 93% of the canola grown in the US is a GM crop, specifically adjusted to withstand spraying with glyphosate-containing Roundup (weed killer). So even before the processing begins, this is a crop that has been genetically altered and sprayed with chemicals that have been implicated in causing cancer.

Words used to describe the processing of canola from seed to oil include "cooking," "hexane solvent," "organic acid," "filtering," and "deodorizing using steam distillation" (28). That's a lot of chemical processing and a lot of heat being applied to unstable, unsaturated fats. Yuck!

Making your own mayo has a mystique about it but it's dead simple if you have a stick blender and a tall container.

Here's the basic recipe but feel free to go crazy with experimentation...

HARDWARE

- Stick immersion blender
- Tall container with a diameter that just holds the blender (usually comes with it). Alternatively, you can use a tall (1 qt/1 l) wide-mouth Mason jar.

INGREDIENTS

- 1 egg
- 1 tbsp lemon juice or apple cider vinegar
- 1 tsp Dijon or other mustard
- ½ tsp salt
- 1 cup oil of choice (extra light olive oil, avocado oil, extra virgin olive oil, liquid coconut oil—lots of possibilities, but use a neutral tasting oil for a regular mayo). Different oils can be combined as well, such as extra light olive oil with some melted bacon fat for a savoury mayo.

Crack egg into blending container, add mustard, salt, and acid of choice. Add oil on top. Place blender in the container right to the bottom and turn on. It will take a few seconds for the whiteness of the emulsified "mayo" to develop. As it does, slowly bring the blender up towards the surface, tipping it slightly to get the liquid oil on the top to incorporate. The sound of the blender will suddenly change as the last of the liquid turns into solid and you're done. Easy peasy!

Transfer to a glass jar for storage in the fridge. Mark with the date if you are someone who forgets things like that. Despite the raw egg, it will be fine for over a week.

NUTRITIONAL INFORMATION:

For 1 tbsp: 100 kcals, 0 g carb, 0 g protein, 11 g fat.

Here's an interesting use for mayo:

Take a piece of fresh or thawed fish filet and brush it thickly with mayo using a basting brush. Mix about a half cup of grated Parmesan cheese with about a teaspoon of Italian seasoning (oregano, basil, garlic powder, etc.) on a plate and press the brushed fish, mayo side down, into the cheese mix to coat it with a thick crust. Place crust side up in a baking dish and cook at 400–425 F for 10–20 minutes (depending on the thickness of your piece of fish—if thawed, it should be about 10 minutes per inch at the thickest part). It's done when it's opaque and flaky all the way through.

Fat Bombs

Fat bombs are small "treats" made of high-fat ingredients to provide a burst of flavour, high satiety value, and no insulin response. They are for use as between-meal snacks, or possibly desserts, when something sweet is called for.

Other than being super tasty, fat bombs are beneficial in several ways. Here are five benefits of fat bombs:

1. **They're satisfying.** Fat bombs, as you would expect, are loaded with (healthy) fats. Because of their high fat content, they can keep you full for hours.

2. **They won't spike your blood sugar.** Because fat bombs are free of added sugars and very low in carbs, they won't spike your blood sugar. Because they are high in fat, they have minimal effect on your insulin levels. If you make them very sweet with non-nutritive sweeteners, they can elicit an insulin response, but most of these recipes are only minimally sweetened, using the natural sweetness of the ingredients to "read" as sweet when you eat them.

3. **They're easy to make.** Most fat bomb recipes only take a few minutes to make.

4. **They're portable.** While you don't want to tote around a big bag of fat bombs in the sweltering heat (especially if they contain a fat like coconut oil that will melt), they're relatively portable when stored in a plastic baggie or small plastic container, especially when the weather isn't too warm.

5. **They satisfy your sweets cravings.** The low-carb diet can sometimes feel like one savoury food after another, so a fat bomb is a nice change of pace from steak and butter.

Find a small plastic or glass container with a volume of 1–2 cups max, preferably with a flat bottom that is approximately 4–5 inches across. Line it with plastic wrap for easy removal of the finished fat bombs.

CINNAMON ALMOND BUTTER FAT BOMBS
- ½ cup almond butter, unsweetened
- ½ cup coconut crème or coconut butter
- 1 heaped tsp cinnamon
- 1–2 pkts of Stevia sweetener or a couple of drops of liquid Stevia, if desired.

In a small glass bowl, microwave the almond butter and coconut cream/butter until softened but not melted. Add the cinnamon. Mash together with a fork. Pour into prepared container, level the top, and chill in the fridge for at least 2 hours until solidified. Lift out of the container using the plastic wrap, place on cutting board, and cut with a sharp knife into ¾–1-inch squares. Store in the fridge for up to a week and eat 2–4 pieces in a serving.

LEMON CHEESECAKE FAT BOMBS
- ½ cup full-fat cream cheese
- ½ cup coconut cream
- Zested rind of ½–1 lemon, depending on how zippy you like it
- 1–2 pkts of Stevia sweetener or a couple of drops of liquid Stevia

In a small glass bowl, soften the cream cheese and coconut cream in the microwave until softened but not melted. Using a fork, mash together with lemon rind and sweetener. Chill in prepared container and cut as indicated in recipe above. These are my favourite!

GINGERSNAP FAT BOMBS
Make them the same as the Cinnamon Almond Butter Fat Bombs but instead of just cinnamon, add 1 heaped teaspoon each of cinnamon, ground ginger, and ground cloves. Chill and cut as usual.

CHOCOLATE ALMOND FAT BOMBS
- ½ cup coconut cream or coconut oil
- ½ cup almond butter or unsweetened peanut butter

- 2 tbsp unsweetened cocoa powder
- 1–2 pkts of Stevia sweetener or a couple of drops of liquid Stevia
- Splash of vanilla extract

In a small glass bowl, soften the coconut cream and almond butter in the microwave then mash in the remaining ingredients using a fork. For added texture, a few slivered almonds or chopped pecans/walnuts could be stirred in after the mixture is smooth. Chill and cut as usual.

Nutritional Information:

All of the above recipes will provide 40–50 kcals per piece, depending on how you cut them, and all will supply 80–85 percent calories from fat.

Chia Seed Fruit Jam

- 1¼ cups fresh or frozen berries, such as strawberries, raspberries, blueberries, or blackberries
- 3 tbsp whole chia seeds
- 1 tsp lemon juice
- 2 tbsp granulated sweetener of choice
- ⅓ cup water

Defrost berries (if necessary) and mash with a fork into a lumpy purée. Add remaining ingredients and mix well. Pour into a jam jar or other small container and refrigerate to set. Chia seeds will expand and soften, thickening and setting the jam. Give them time—they are crunchy until fully softened. Once set, stir well again and enjoy.

NUTRITIONAL INFORMATION:

Portion: one tablespoon

25 kcals, 1 g of net carbs. This will vary depending on fruit used.

Mason Jar Ice Cream

This is another of the "keto treats" that's very sweet and can meet a need but should be an occasional event. If you're feeling hungry but a bit nauseous, even a few teaspoons of this ice cream, taken in tiny bites, can soothe the mouth and stomach. It freezes harder than regular ice cream, but if you take it out and let it sit on the counter for a few minutes, you can scrape up small spoonfuls of creamy deliciousness. Built-in portion control.

Start with a 2 cup (500 ml) wide mouth Mason jar and lid. This can be made in a plastic container but with all the shaking involved, a screw-on lid is safest.

INGREDIENTS
- 1 cup heavy whipping cream
- 2–3 tbsp monk fruit/erythritol blend
- 1 tsp vanilla extract

That's all you need for the basic vanilla ice cream. Optional add-ins could be any of the following, or any combination of the following:
- ¼ tsp cinnamon
- 2 tbsp chopped pecans
- 2 tbsp coconut flakes
- 2 tbsp Lily's dark chocolate chips or similarly low-carb chocolate chunks
- Maple extract or rum extract in place of the vanilla
- ½–1 tbsp cocoa powder
- 1 tsp or more instant coffee (unsweetened)

Screw the lid on tightly and shake the contents vigorously for 5 minutes or so until the cream has almost doubled in size. Place the jar in the freezer for a minimum of 3 hours. If you have used chunky contents such as nuts or chocolate chips, they will all sink to the bottom so pull the jar out after 2 hours or so and stir up the half-frozen contents if you care about even distribution. I never worry. The top half of the jar is a different ice cream experience than the bottom half of the jar. It's like digging for buried treasure!

NUTRITION INFORMATION (PER ¼ RECIPE OF THE BASIC VANILLA)
210 kcals, 2 g protein, 2 g net carbs, 21 g fat.

Appendix 1
The Quick and Dirty Guide

This guide is meant to give you the basic protocol without any explanations or anecdotes. Just the facts, ma'am...

Fasting for Chemotherapy

For intermittent chemotherapy (every 2–3 weeks):

Measure out 36 hours pre-chemo.

Measure out 24–30 hours after chemo.

This is your fasting period. Adjust according to your chemo schedule.

PREPARATION:

Have available 500–750 ml minimum of bone broth. Defrost it if necessary so it's ready to go.

Plan out how to have coffee, tea, water/soda water, and bone broth available and with you at all times. You'll need water bottles, thermal cups, thermos flasks.

Day 1 – Finish eating a satisfying supper in the evening, then take no additional solid food or caloric beverages after that. Tea/herbal tea/water only.

Day 2 – Black coffee (add up to 1 teaspoon of heavy cream if absolutely necessary—measure it!), black, green, or herbal tea, water, soda water.

Use bone broth as a meal replacer for lunch and supper. Serve hot, sip slowly.

If you feel overwhelmed by hunger sensations, use additional bone broth with salt to ride it out.

Day 3 – Chemo Day. Continue with allowed fluids, making sure that you have a clear plan for having them with you throughout your chemo visit. Have your support person refill them for you as necessary. Drink lots of water. If nausea becomes an issue, stick with water or water with a bit of real lemon juice.

Day 4 – First day post chemo. Continue with allowed fluids, using bone broth if desired to replace lunch. Plan for a modest supper that really appeals to you. Avoid highly spicy or fatty foods for this first meal._

Constipation Protocol

Remember that constipation is defined by the hardness of your stool, not by the size or frequency. You don't have to go every day but it should be soft and easy to pass when you do go. Establish the daily anti-constipation practice of using psyllium or flax meal (or a combination) for stool bulking and to keep stools soft but solid. Both are low-carb and keto-compliant. See my recipe for Magic Keto Flax/Psyllium Bread for Constipation Relief for a tasty way to supplement with these fibre sources. Start with two slices per day and adjust to the amount that keeps you fairly regular.

Discuss any regular use of medications with your medical team. Restoralax/Lax-A-Day (polyethylene glycol) works by attracting water into the large bowel, where it keeps stools soft. Much gentler than the stimulant-type laxatives which irritate the gut into cramping and pushing out stool. It's a powder that you stir into liquid, making it easy to take during the chemo fast.

Day 1 – Have your regular intake of keto flax bread before your eating cut-off time.

Day 2 – Fluids only. You can add a serving of Restoralax in the evening before chemo if needed.

Day 3 – Chemo Day. Have a serving of Restoralax in the evening after chemo.

Day 4 – Have a serving of your Magic Keto Flax Bread in the evening either with or after your fast-breaking supper meal.

Day 5 onward – Have a serving of Magic Keto Flax Bread every day. Monitor yourself —don't let the constipation get ahead of you.

Keto Diet in 14 Easy Steps

- **Remove all sugar and sugar-containing foods** from your diet. Everything! This includes honey, maple syrup, agave syrup, jams, most sweet condiments like BBQ sauce or relishes.
- **Remove all foods containing industrial seed oils** from your diet. That's soybean oil, corn oil, canola oil, margarine, shortening. Make your own mayo.
- **Remove all wheat and grain foods** from your diet. That's bread, pasta, rice, cookies, deep-fried snack foods, cakes, donuts. Also, highly starchy vegetables, such as potatoes and most root vegetables (carrots, rutabagas, beets).
- **Eat a moderate meat/fish/poultry/egg** serving at every meal. No breading or sweet sauces.
- **Eat a variety of brightly coloured vegetables.** Most vegetables that grow above ground, with the exception of corn, are acceptable. These can be raw, steamed, sautéed, spiralized, puréed—whatever works.
- **Eat sparingly of dark berries** (fresh or frozen)—blueberries, strawberries, raspberries—max ½ cup per day.
- **Use only full-fat dairy products.** Heavy whipping cream, full-fat sour cream, full-fat cheeses, full-fat cream cheese, butter. Try to use dairy products as condiments, not the main event.
- **Unsweetened nut milks can be used for beverage or cooking if desired.** Do not use soy milk. These are highly processed and minimally nutritious. Don't use them unless you really need to.

- **Add healthy fats to every meal**. These are butter, olive oil, home-made healthy oil mayo, pure nut butters, avocado, olives, ghee, coconut oil. Fat is your friend. Use it generously.
- **Eat enough at each meal to be satiated.** Not stuffed but full and happy. Ideally 2–3 meals per day and no snacks.
- **Snack only when absolutely necessary.** Use nuts, cheese, or meat for snacks. Fat bombs if you need something sweet but not as a regular event.
- **Avoid artificial sweeteners.** Try to only use Stevia, monk fruit, or erythritol. And only as little as possible. Eating large quantities of "keto baking," stimulating the sweet taste receptors, can stimulate insulin release.
- **Drink lots of noncaloric fluids.** Water, coffee, tea, green or herbal teas, or soda water without sweetness. Don't drink commercial diet sodas sweetened with industrial sweeteners. Save Stevia-sweetened sodas (e.g. Zevia) for a rare treat.
- **Drink minimal alcoholic beverages.** Avoid beer, sweet wines, most cocktails. A single glass of a dry red wine or a pure liquor (not liqueur!) occasionally: Vodka, rum, whiskey, gin. Alone over ice or in a sugar-free cocktail.

Appendix 2
The Evidence / Research

Numbered Citations

1. Vernieri, C., Casola, S., Foiani, M., Pietrantonio, F., de Braud, F., & Longo, V. (2016). Targeting Cancer Metabolism: Dietary and Pharmacologic Interventions. *Cancer Discovery, 6*(12), 1315–33. https://doi.org/10.1158/2159-8290.CD-16-0615
2. Thanh, N. X., Wanke, M., & McGeachy, L. (2013). Wait time from primary to specialty care: a trend analysis from Edmonton, Canada. *Healthcare policy = Politiques de Santé, 8*(4), 35–44.
3. Vander Heiden, M. G., Cantley, L. C., & Thompson, C. B. (2009). Understanding the Warburg effect: the metabolic requirements of cell proliferation. *Science (New York, N.Y.), 324*(5930), 1029–33. https://doi.org/10.1126/science.1160809
4. Kearns C.E., Schmidt L.A., & Glantz S.A. (2016). Sugar Industry and Coronary Heart Disease Research: A Historical Analysis of Internal Industry Documents. *JAMA Intern Med., 176*(11),1680–85. doi:10.1001/jamainternmed.2016.5394
5. van Niekerk, G., Hattingh, S. M., & Engelbrecht, A. M. (2016). Enhanced Therapeutic Efficacy in Cancer Patients by Short-term Fasting: The Autophagy Connection. *Frontiers in Oncology, 6*(242). https://doi.org/10.3389/fonc.2016.00242
6. Safdie, F. M., Dorff, T., Quinn, D., Fontana, L., Wei, M., Lee, C., Cohen, P., & Longo, V. D. (2009). Fasting and cancer treatment in humans: A case series report. *Aging, 1*(12), 988–1007. https://doi.org/10.18632/aging.100114
7. Seyfried, T. N., Yu, G., Maroon, J. C., & D'Agostino, D. P.

(2017). Press-pulse: a novel therapeutic strategy for the metabolic management of cancer. *Nutrition & Metabolism, 14*(19). https://doi.org/10.1186/s12986-017-0178-2

8. Champ, C. E., Palmer, J. D., Volek, J. S., Werner-Wasik, M., Andrews, D. W., Evans, J. J., Glass, J., Kim, L., & Shi, W. (2014). Targeting metabolism with a ketogenic diet during the treatment of glioblastoma multiforme. *Journal of Neuro-oncology, 117*(1), 125–31. https://doi.org/10.1007/s11060-014-1362-0

9. Oke, J. L., O'Sullivan, J. W., Perera, R., & Nicholson, B. D. (2018). The mapping of cancer incidence and mortality trends in the UK from 1980–2013 reveals a potential for overdiagnosis. *Scientific Reports, 8*(1), 14663. https://doi.org/10.1038/s41598-018-32844-x

10. Weir, H. K., Thompson, T. D., Soman, A., Møller, B., & Leadbetter, S. (2015). The past, present, and future of cancer incidence in the United States: 1975 through 2020. *Cancer, 121*(11), 1827–37. https://doi.org/10.1002/cncr.29258

11. https://www.nytimes.com/2016/05/15/magazine/warburg-effect-an-old-idea-revived-starve-cancer-to-death.html

12. Pollan, Michael. (2008). *In Defense of Food: An Eater's Manifesto.* New York: Penguin Press.

13. http://www.ers.usda.gov/data-products/adoption-of-genetically-engineered-crops-in-the-us/recent-trends-in-ge-adoption.aspx

14. https://www.centerforfoodsafety.org/issues/311/ge-foods/about-ge-foods

15. Ben-Dor, M. & Gopher, A. & Hershkovitz, I. & Barkai, R. (2011). Man the Fat Hunter: The Demise of Homo erectus and the Emergence of a New Hominin Lineage in the Middle Pleistocene (ca. 400 kyr) Levant. *PLOS ONE.* 6. e28689. 10.1371/journal.pone.0028689.

16. Okada, H., Kuhn, C., Feillet, H., & Bach, J. F. (2010). The 'hygiene hypothesis' for autoimmune and allergic diseases: an update. *Clinical and Experimental Immunology, 160*(1), 1–9. https://doi.org/10.1111/j.1365-2249.2010.04139.x

17. https://www.sciencemag.org/news/2020/02/cutting-edge-crispr-gene-editing-appears-safe-three-cancer-patients

18. Schmitt, M. W., Prindle, M. J., & Loeb, L. A. (2012). Implications of genetic heterogeneity in cancer. *Annals of the New York Academy of Sciences, 1267*(110–16). https://doi.org/10.1111/j.1749-6632.2012.06590.x

19. Bauersfeld, S. P., Kessler, C. S., Wischnewsky, M., Jaensch, A., Steckhan, N., Stange, R., Kunz, B., Brückner, B., Sehouli, J., & Michalsen, A. (2018). The effects of short-term fasting on quality of life and tolerance to chemotherapy in patients with breast and ovarian cancer: a randomized cross-over pilot study. *BMC Cancer, 18*(1), 476. https://doi.org/10.1186/s12885-018-4353-2

20. http://chemocare.com/

21. Caccialanza, R., Cereda, E., De Lorenzo, F., Farina, G., Pedrazzoli, P., & AIOM-SINPE-FAVO Working Group (2018). To fast, or not to fast before chemotherapy, that is the question. *BMC Cancer, 18*(1), 337. https://doi.org/10.1186/s12885-018-4245-5

22. Sharma, A., Madaan, V., & Petty, F. D. (2006). Exercise for mental health. *Primary Care Companion to the Journal of Clinical Psychiatry, 8*(2), 106. https://doi.org/10.4088/pcc.v08n0208a

23. Daniel, Y. T. Fong, J.W.C.H., Bryant, P. H. Hui, Antoinette M. Lee, Duncan, J. Macfarlane, Sharron S. K. Leung, Ester Cerin, Wynnie Y. Y. Chan, Ivy P. F. Leung, Sharon H. S. Lam, Aliki J. Taylor, Kar-keung Cheng, (2012). Physical activity for cancer survivors: Meta analysis of randomised controlled trials. *British Medical Journal, 344*(70).

24. Ruud Knols, N.K.A., Uebelhart, D., Fransen, J., & and Aufdemkampe, G. (2005). Physical exercise in cancer patients during and after medical treatment: A systematic review of randomized and controlled clinical trials. *Journal of Clinical Oncology, 23*(16), 3830–42.

25. Liśkiewicz, A. D., Kasprowska, D., Wojakowska, A., Polański, K., Lewin-Kowalik, J., Kotulska, K., & Jędrzejowska-Szypułka, H. (2016). Long-term High Fat Ketogenic Diet Promotes Renal Tumor Growth in a Rat Model of Tuberous Sclerosis. *Scientific Reports, 6*, 21807. https://doi.org/10.1038/srep21807

26. Liśkiewicz, A. D., Kasprowska, D., Wojakowska, A., Polański,

K., Lewin-Kowalik, J., Kotulska, K., & Jędrzejowska-Szypułka, H. (2016). Long-term High Fat Ketogenic Diet Promotes Renal Tumor Growth in a Rat Model of Tuberous Sclerosis. *Scientific Reports, 6,* 21807. https://doi.org/10.1038/srep21807

27. Cheng, C. W., Adams, G. B., Perin, L., Wei, M., Zhou, X., Lam, B. S., Da Sacco, S., Mirisola, M., Quinn, D. I., Dorff, T. B., Kopchick, J. J., & Longo, V. D. (2014). Prolonged fasting reduces IGF-1/PKA to promote hematopoietic-stem-cell-based regeneration and reverse immunosuppression. *Cell Stem Cell, 14*(6), 810–23. https://doi.org/10.1016/j.stem.2014.04.014

28. https://www.canolacouncil.org/oil-and-meal/what-is-canola/how-canola-is-processed/steps-in-oil-and-meal-processing/

29. Maurer, T., von Grundherr, J., Patra. S., *et al* (2020). An exercise and nutrition intervention for ovarian cancer patients during and after first-line chemotherapy (BENITA study): a randomized controlled pilot trial *International Journal of Gynecologic Cancer, 30* 541–45.

30. von Haehling, S., & Anker, S. D. (2014). Prevalence, incidence and clinical impact of cachexia: facts and numbers-update 2014. *Journal of Cachexia, Sarcopenia and Muscle, 5*(4), 261–63. https://doi.org/10.1007/s13539-014-0164-8

31. Catenacci, V. A., Pan, Z., Ostendorf, D., Brannon, S., Gozansky, W. S., Mattson, M. P., Martin, B., MacLean, P. S., Melanson, E. L., & Troy Donahoo, W. (2016). A randomized pilot study comparing zero-calorie alternate-day fasting to daily caloric restriction in adults with obesity. *Obesity (Silver Spring, Md.), 24*(9), 1874–83. https://doi.org/10.1002/oby.21581

32. Raffaghello, L., Lee, C., Safdie, F. M., Wei, M., Madia, F., Bianchi, G., & Longo, V. D. (2008). Starvation-dependent differential stress resistance protects normal but not cancer cells against high-dose chemotherapy. *Proceedings of the National Academy of Sciences of the United States of America, 105*(24), 8215–20. https://doi.org/10.1073/pnas.0708100105

Additional Research Articles

Fasting

"Why do women fast during breast cancer chemotherapy? A qualitative study of the patient experience"
https://www.ncbi.nlm.nih.gov/pubmed/30825263

"Fasting and cancer treatment in humans: A case series report"
https://www.ncbi.nlm.nih.gov/pubmed/20157582

"When less may be more: Calorie restriction and response to cancer therapy"
https://www.ncbi.nlm.nih.gov/pubmed/28539118

"Safety and feasibility of fasting in combination with platinum-based chemotherapy"
https://www.ncbi.nlm.nih.gov/pubmed/27282289

"Fasting cycles retard growth of tumors and sensitize a range of cancer cell types to chemotherapy"
https://www.ncbi.nlm.nih.gov/pubmed/22323820

"The effects of short-term fasting on tolerance to (neo) adjuvant chemotherapy in HER2-negative breast cancer patients: a randomized pilot study"
https://www.ncbi.nlm.nih.gov/pubmed/26438237

"Enhanced therapeutic efficacy in cancer patients by short-term fasting: The autophagy connection"
https://www.ncbi.nlm.nih.gov/pubmed/27896219

"The effects of short-term fasting on quality of life and tolerance to chemotherapy in patients with breast and ovarian cancer: A randomized crossover pilot study"
https://www.ncbi.nlm.nih.gov/pubmed/29699509

"Fasting cycles potentiate the efficacy of gemcitabine treatment in in vitro and in vivo pancreatic cancer models"
https://www.ncbi.nlm.nih.gov/pubmed/26176887

"Fasting induces anti-Warburg effect that increases respiration but reduces ATP-synthesis to promote apoptosis in colon cancer models"
https://www.ncbi.nlm.nih.gov/pubmed/25909219

"Fasting: starving cancer"
https://www.ncbi.nlm.nih.gov/pubmed/28368246

"Selectively starving cancer cells through dietary manipulation: Methods and clinical implications."
https://www.ncbi.nlm.nih.gov/pubmed/23837760

"Fasting regulates EGR1 and protects from glucose- and dexamethasone-dependent sensitization to chemotherapy"
https://www.ncbi.nlm.nih.gov/pubmed/28358805

"Starvation based differential chemotherapy: A novel approach for cancer treatment"
https://www.ncbi.nlm.nih.gov/pubmed/25584154

"Fasting and differential chemotherapy protection in patients"
https://www.ncbi.nlm.nih.gov/pubmed/21088487

"Autophagy and intermittent fasting: The connection for cancer therapy?"
https://www.ncbi.nlm.nih.gov/pubmed/30540126

"Starvation-dependent differential stress resistance protects normal but not cancer cells against high-dose chemotherapy"
https://www.ncbi.nlm.nih.gov/pubmed/18378900

"Reduced levels of IGF-I mediate differential protection of normal and cancer cells in response to fasting and improve chemotherapeutic index" https://www.ncbi.nlm.nih.gov/pubmed/20145127

"Pre-treatment with alternate day modified fast will permit higher dose and frequency of cancer chemotherapy and better cure rates"
https://www.ncbi.nlm.nih.gov/pubmed/19135806

Ketogenic Diets
"The ketogenic diet is an effective adjuvant to radiation therapy for the treatment of malignant glioma"
https://www.ncbi.nlm.nih.gov/pubmed/22563484

"Targeting metabolism with a ketogenic diet during the treatment of glioblastoma multiforme"
https://www.ncbi.nlm.nih.gov/pubmed/24442482

"Calories and carcinogenesis: Lessons learned from 30 years of calorie restriction research"
https://www.ncbi.nlm.nih.gov/pubmed/19969554

"Antitumor effects of ketogenic diets in mice: A meta-analysis"
https://www.ncbi.nlm.nih.gov/pubmed/27159218

"Beneficial effects of ketogenic diets for cancer patients: A realist review with focus on evidence and confirmation"
https://www.ncbi.nlm.nih.gov/pubmed/28653283

"Effects of a ketogenic diet on the quality of life in 16 patients with advanced cancer: A pilot trial"
https://nutritionandmetabolism.biomedcentral.com/articles/10.1186/1743-7075-8-54

"A nutritional perspective of ketogenic diet in cancer: A narrative review"
https://www.ncbi.nlm.nih.gov/pubmed/28366810

"Ketogenic diets in medical oncology: A systematic review with focus on clinical outcomes"
https://www.ncbi.nlm.nih.gov/pubmed/31927631

"Insulin enhances migration and invasion in prostate cancer cells by up-regulation of FOXC2"
https://www.ncbi.nlm.nih.gov/pubmed/31379747

"Targeting glucose metabolism to enhance immunotherapy: Emerging evidence on intermittent fasting and calorie restriction mimetics"
https://www.ncbi.nlm.nih.gov/pubmed/31293576

"Growth of human gastric cancer cells in nude mice is delayed by a ketogenic diet supplemented with omega-3 fatty acids and medium-chain triglycerides"
https://www.ncbi.nlm.nih.gov/pubmed/18447912

"Postoperative serum metabolites of patients on a low carbohydrate ketogenic diet after pancreatectomy for pancreatobiliary cancer: A nontargeted metabolomics pilot study."
https://www.ncbi.nlm.nih.gov/pubmed/31727967

Poff, A. M., Ari, C., Arnold, P., Seyfried, T. N., & D'Agostino, D. P. (2014). "Ketone supplementation decreases tumor cell viability and prolongs survival of mice with metastatic cancer. International Journal of Cancer", 135(7), 1711–20
https://doi.org/10.1002/ijc.28809

Cancer and Autophagy

"Role of autophagy in cancer prevention"
https://www.ncbi.nlm.nih.gov/pmc/articles/PMC3136921/

Books and Blogs

Most of these books have been instrumental in shaping my understanding of low-carb nutrition, fasting, and the metabolic nature of cancer. As books written for the public, they take the science of the academic journals and make it accessible for everyone. Some are quite in-depth, some are more practically oriented. Most are also available on Kindle or as audiobooks. Many of these authors have websites, blogs, YouTube channels, or podcasts where you can follow them for the latest developments in the field of nutrition, cancer, fasting, and nutritional health. Just search their names to find their latest work.

Cancer

Keto for Cancer: Ketogenic Metabolic Therapy as a Targeted Nutritional Strategy, Miriam Kalamian, Chelsea Green Publishing; 1st edition (2017).

The Metabolic Approach to Cancer: Integrating Deep Nutrition, the Ketogenic Diet, and Nontoxic Bio-Individualized Therapies, Dr. Nasha Winters and Jess Higgins Kelley, Chelsea Green Publishing (2017).

Tripping over the Truth: How the Metabolic Theory of Cancer Is Overturning One of Medicine's Most Entrenched Paradigms, Travis Christofferson, Chelsea Green Publishing (2017).

Radical Remission: Surviving Cancer Against All Odds, Dr. Kelly A. Turner PhD, HarperOne (2014).

Cancer as a Metabolic Disease: On the Origin, Management, and Prevention of Cancer, Thomas Seyfried, Wiley (2012).

Nutrition history: how we got so messed up

The Big Fat Surprise: Why Butter, Meat and Cheese Belong in a Healthy Diet, Nina Teicholz, Simon & Schuster; Reprint edition (2015).

Death by Food Pyramid: How Shoddy Science, Sketchy Politics and Shady Special Interests Have Ruined Our Health, Denise Minger, Primal Nutrition, Inc.; 1st edition (2014).

Good Calories, Bad Calories: Fats, Carbs, and the Controversial Science of Diet and Health, Gary Taubes, Anchor; Reprint edition (2008).

Fasting

The Complete Guide to Fasting: Heal Your Body Through Intermittent, Alternate-Day, and Extended Fasting, Dr. Jason Fung and Jimmy Moore, Victory Belt Publishing; 1st edition (2016).

Life in the Fasting Lane: How to Make Intermittent Fasting a Lifestyle—and Reap the Benefits of Weight Loss and Better Health, Dr Jason Fung, Eve Mayer and Megan Ramos, Harper Wave; 1st edition (2020).

Low carbohydrate healthy fats diet and lifestyle

Why We Get Fat: And What to Do About It, Gary Taubes, Anchor; Reprint edition (2011).

The Primal Blueprint, Mark Sisson, Primal Nutrition, Inc.; Fourth Edition (2019).

The Obesity Code: Unlocking the Secrets of Weight Loss, Jason Fung, Greystone Books; 1st edition (2016).

The Diabetes Code: Prevent and Reverse Type 2 Diabetes Naturally, Jason Fung, Greystone Books; 1st edition (2018).

The Case Against Sugar Gary Taubes, Anchor; Reprint edition (2017).

The Keto Reset Diet: Reboot Your Metabolism in 21 Days and Burn Fat Forever, Mark Sisson, Harmony; 1st edition (2017).

Food Addictions

Food Junkies: The Truth About Food Addiction, Vera Tarman, Dundurn; 1st edition (2014).

Real Food

In Defense of Food: An Eater's Manifesto, Michael Pollan, Penguin Books; 1st edition (2009).

Undoctored: How You Can Seize Control of Your Health and Become Smarter Than Your Doctor, William Davis MD, Collins (2017).
Deep Nutrition: Why Your Genes Need Traditional Food, Catherine Shanahan, M.D, Flatiron Books; Reprint edition (2018).
The Longevity Diet: Slow Aging, Fight Disease, Optimize Weight, Valter Longo, Avery (2019).